Nurturing the Family

A DOULA'S GUIDE TO SUPPORTING NEW PARENTS

Second Edition

Updated for the changing landscape of parenting

JACQUELINE KELLEHER

Praeclarus Press, LLC
©2020 Jacqueline Kelleher. All rights reserved.

www.PraeclarusPress.com

Praeclarus Press, LLC
2504 Sweetgum Lane
Amarillo, Texas 79124 USA
806-367-9950
www.PraeclarusPress.com

DISCLAIMER
The information contained in this publication is advisory only and is not intended to replace sound clinical judgment or individualized patient care. The author disclaims all warranties, whether expressed or implied, including any warranty as the quality, accuracy, safety, or suitability of this information for any particular purpose.

ISBN: 978-1-946665-43-0

Cover Design: Chris Dietrich
Developmental Editing: Kathleen Kendall-Tackett
Copyediting: Chris Tackett
Layout & Design: Nelly Murariu

For my babies
Ryan, Lauren, and Rachel

... and now this Second Edition is for James, our caboose.

Contents

Other Voices for Professional Doulas

On the Experiences and Support Needs of Families

The Why and the How
of Doula Support

How to Use This Book

This book is a primer for professionals, family members, and others who doula families through their early parenting experiences. In recent years, we have come to use the word doula as a verb; "to doula" is to serve as a source of nurture and support for any person, in any situation. Family members, friends, social workers, and nurses can all serve as doulas. Formal training is not required. In these pages, you will find actionable practices and support approaches to augment your skills within existing roles.

This book is not intended to stand on its own for professional doulas. We are fortunate recipients of an ever-growing bounty of writings and organizations to educate us on the specifics of topics to include breastfeeding, the newborn, perinatal mental health, and much more. Most of these underscore the importance of support, yet there is little focus on how to create a competent support community. This book is created to address that need. Effective support of growing families requires a diversity of both community and knowledge. Time and experience make clear that this is a field that reaches into all areas of life. The doula, therefore, requires education specifically focused on the art of support. The information here is actionable by any person who will be "doula-ing" a family through the weeks postpartum. For the aspiring professional, *Nurturing the Family* can be read either before or after attending doula training, but not in place of one. Topics are deliberately brief. Their purpose is to offer an introduction, spark enthusiasm, and serve as a springboard toward further exploration. Topics in *Other Voices* topics go into more depth, are considerably longer, and are written by experts within related areas of specialization.

Why Do We Need Doulas?

It may be surprising to learn that what some consider the *modern* experiences of new families may not be shared by the rest of the world. In fact, one can easily argue that modern birth traditions, which focus mostly on the purchasing of gifts, are inadequate compared with those of more traditional cultures. It seems that many babies have a car seat, stroller, swing, bouncy seat, toys, and books. Their parents, however, are often unprepared and unsupported. Most babies are born in hospitals, to parents who may or may not have education or experience in infant care. The mother and baby remain in the hospital for just a day or two, and then the family goes home. The door closes, and the support ends. With the exception of well-baby visits to the pediatrician, or the rare one or two visits from a visiting nurse, parents have no guarantee of parenting mentorship or support to help them through the early months while they recover and adapt.

In contrast, many non-industrial nations practice a period of isolation or *cushioning* of the new mother and her baby. During this time, the mother is frequently isolated from the rest of the community. Traditions during this time include massage of the mother with special herbs and oils, the cooking of foods considered especially healing for the mother, and wrapping of the mother's head. The mother is not expected to care for others or perform any of her regular responsibilities. The duration of "cushioning" varies but is usually between eight and forty days.

Anthropologists studying these traditions have recognized a disappointing trend. Just as our rainforests are disappearing, the number of traditional societies maintaining the purity of their customs is decreasing. In many parts of the world, birth and early parenting are being brought closer to "modern living." The potential of life-saving technology comes with the cost of women giving birth in hospitals, to which they need to travel. In doing so, they forfeit some of their familial and community support. Traditional common wisdom in basic aspects of life to include labor support, nursing, infant soothing, and mother care are lost to hospital protocols, the formula industry, and mass campaigns that do not consider culture and individuality.

Many modern countries practice almost no traditions to welcome the woman in her new carnation, mother, back to the community. Mothers birth in a setting that is often focused on the individual parts (uterus, fetus, vagina, breast) rather than the whole person. Separation from the baby works in conflict with the expectations of the human body. Research consistently concludes that mothers and babies belong together, yet powerful industries modify our social expectations to focus on apparatus to take the place of the parent-newborn relationship rather than supporting the relationship itself.

Mothers give birth using medication and often surgically. Babies are brought to nurseries for screening, bathing, and ostensibly to increase the mother's rest. Hospital staff may be wonderfully supportive and instructive, or they may not. That wonderfully supportive nurse can't attend every birth. Perhaps the lactation consultant isn't there on the weekend. Or it's a holiday. Perhaps the family gets to spend 20 or even 30 minutes with this supportive staff person during their entire hospital stay. Then this family is released to their home, where the challenge repeats. There may be knowledgeable, supportive family members and community waiting to support them. Alternatively, there could be family members waiting, but not at all supportive. Or there may be no support at all. Googling and online communities may be sources of mentorship and support, but they may also be a source of misinformation. There is an absence of tailoring support to the particular personalities and needs of this one family. In addition, our family leave policies are an underlying cause of many early parenting choices, to include inductions, repeat cesareans, and whether to breastfeed.

Given the lack of effective systems to provide individualized support, it's a wonder that families thrive, but they do. The question is at what cost?

You Can Do This

You can do this. People need YOU, for precisely who you are and what you have to offer them. You aren't perfect, but guess what? They aren't looking for perfect. You don't know everything and never will. You won't be the perfect match for everyone, and that is just fine.

There's something about you, something that people will be drawn to and click with. Maybe it's your gentle spirit. Maybe it's your fire, your passion. Your attentiveness. Your intelligence. Your knowledge. Your quirkiness. Your resources. Your eye contact. Maybe you look like them. Maybe you sound like them. Maybe you remind them of home. Whatever it is, people will need you.

Don't let insecurities hold you back. Don't worry if you're not yet feeling the expert. Ours is a timeless role. If you want the best for this family, if you bring your best each and every time, you are what they need. If you bring your willing heart and hands to each visit, you will make a difference. If your goal is to listen rather than to share. If you believe in this family. Sound familiar? If so, you are already a doula. Now, let's begin.

About Me

You may wonder about who I am and what qualifies me to offer my opinions on the needs of growing families. When I wrote the First Edition of *Nurturing the Family*, I had been a doula for years, was a birth doula trainer, and had a degree in education. I had also recently taken on the task of deeply investigating research on the subject as part of co-creating DONA's (later to become DONA International) postpartum doula certification program. I knew quite a bit, had a respected voice in the doula community, and was eager to share what I had learned.

Interestingly, from today's vantage point, that time feels like the beginning. My doula life really took off from that point. I taught hundreds of doula trainings, mostly in the U.S., but some outside of it. That meant opportunities to offer what I had learned to a diversity of people. More important was all that those people had to offer me. My students were effective educators, spurring me to further my own understanding of what people need to thrive. I served as program mentor for DONA's postpartum certification program for 15 years, which allowed me to learn through working relationships with experts in the field. Mentoring doulas and doula trainers offered additional insights. I have benefitted from so many teachers!

In 2007, I opened BirthMark, a Philadelphia-area community center for growing families. For five years, I doula-ed core groups of families who cycled in during pregnancy and often stayed for the first year or longer. I did this through daily educational offerings and support groups. Breastfeeding support groups, early parenting groups, sleep groups, loss and grief groups—six days a week, I was immersed in my support role. It was trial by fire, and it was intense.

Accountability was a motivator in being certain of my resources and information. The maternity nurse makes their recommendations and moves on to the next patient; if parents find their advice to be unhelpful or even disruptive, there is almost no way to offer feedback to that individual days or even weeks later. In my situation, the door was always open. I had a constant, sometimes dizzying feedback loop from the stream of parents who frequented BirthMark. It was here that I learned practicality. What we read in books or are told in classes is theory; application of those concepts will have varied results because families and individuals vary. BirthMark underscored the flexibility that my early support years had suggested.

When I wrote my First Edition, it seemed I knew so much. Today, I feel differently. I have thousands of hours of additional support experience, and they have shaped me. I have countless additional doula training and mentoring experiences, and those have also shaped me. I offer wisdom accrued from the families and doulas who have been my teachers. If you're like me, you may feel a driving need to know more; the more I know, the more I'm aware of what needs further exploration. If these writings leave you aching for the next step, I'll consider this edition a success.

Nurturing the Doula Within

"Hi, I'm Jackie. I'm going to be your doula-ing doula." You may already have a doula mentor, and hopefully, you will have many more as you evolve within your role. Some people come to doula work with a desire to lead and provide instruction. While there are aspects of what we offer that require these skills, ours is more of a coming alongside role. We lead by following—following the style, preferences, and pace of our clients. This means that rather than telling our clients what to do, we educate them on options and help them feel their way to the option that fits their family.

Heads up; I'm going to do the same thing with you. For us, it means that I'm not going to provide you with a formula for setting up your business or practice. There are too many factors to possibly offer a cookie-cutter approach. Personality, geography, target client-base, and areas of specialty all come into play. It quickly becomes plain that we can't all offer the same thing. Nor should we! Isn't it great to consider that there's just the right doula out there for each family?

I wish you many mentors and many voices to draw upon as you move forward. I want my voice to be the one to plant the seed of being gentle with yourself. With being flexible. With allowing space to grow and evolve. Take risks. Adapt. These are the spaces in which real learning happens.

We Are All Unique

In writing this book, there are topics that, for me, present themselves as top priorities; topics like culture, oppression, and disability. Concepts that themselves are deserving of entire books and courses of study, and that's what I'm recommending. Take the time to understand more about people who are less like you—less like you in any of the ways. There are experts who can speak to these topics with so much more fluency and efficacy than I, so I've decided to say this:

We are all unique. You'll note that concept is woven throughout this book. Don't expect any one approach to work with everyone. Every family is unique; every person within that family is also unique. So is every individual who doulas a family. As a result, your experience in supporting families should be varied. Bring fresh eyes and a fresh mindset to each experience, recognizing that every family that you support has its own culture, and respect it. Recognize that every single person has their gifts and their challenges, including yourself. Learn from others. Adapt.

Glossary

We begin our support of growing families with an acknowledgment that the word "family" has no single definition. In recognition of the great diversity of families, the glossary below contains definitions of roles that may not yet be familiar to the reader. It also contains the manner in which certain words will be intended to be interpreted within the pages of this book, and solely there.

Family   One or more adults parenting one or more children.

Mother   A parent who identifies as a woman.

Father   A parent who identifies as a man.

Parent   A person of any gender identification who is a primary caregiver.

Partner   A person of any gender identification who is in a committed relationship with a parent. Often parents, but in some cases not.

Birthing Parent   The person who will give birth to a baby. Not all birthing parents identify as mothers. This would be the case with a transgender man who chooses to carry a baby.

Pronouns   Not all doulas are women. Not all people identify with the gender their anatomy provides them with. At times in this book, you will find the pronouns *they* or *them*. This is not an error; it is an acknowledgement of diversity.

The Art of
Supporting New Families

Self-Care While Caregiving

I'm placing this topic way up here at the top because that's where it needs to live—at the top of your consciousness. Burying it further down might imply that you should do the same, and that is not the message that I want to send. Caregiving is energizing and heartwarming, and at the same time, it can be depleting. The skills required to practice active, intentional support—removing your own story, careful consideration of actions and words, staying within boundaries—are all hard work.

Just as expectant parents may anticipate diaper changing and physical care of the baby to be the challenging aspects of baby-care, doula support holds its surprises as well. You'll experience the expected fulfilled fatigue that comes with a job well done, and weeks and even months go by feeling very manageable. Eventually, doula-ing may feel draining at a deeper level. Feeling emotionally intertwined can keep your mind whirling long after you return home. Navigating challenging family dynamics and having the hard conversations thoughtfully and intentionally can feel like the equivalent of emotional calisthenics. Puddle sit for long enough, and you may be ready to create a puddle of your own when you get home.

It becomes clear that the doula needs to exercise self-care on an ongoing basis. Just as it's ideal for expecting parents to create a postpartum plan, invest your time and thought in a self-care plan. Ask yourself,

✓ What can I do on a daily or ongoing basis to care for myself? What are my most basic needs?

✓ What triggers or buttons am I aware of? Have I developed strategies around them?

✓ What will feel nurturing to me during stressful times—while I am with a family? After I have returned home?

✓ Who are my personal support people? Who will I turn to for my own physical and emotional needs?

During or after a new or challenging time with a family, journal about the experience and create a script to remind yourself of strategies that helped in this situation, as well as any proactive communication skills or boundaries that might ease future situations. Create a basket of cues for self-nurture, and take it out and use it often. Each person's needs for self-care are different and often evolve, so expect the contents to change over time.

Here are some ideas to get you started: A journal, essential oils, running shorts, names and numbers of friends to call, a gift card to a favorite meal, a list of hikes, the number of a massage therapist, or a list of books you've been wanting to read. It's okay if your basket doesn't have much in the way of contents to begin with, or perhaps ever. You know yourself. The message here is to make and keep self-care as a priority.

The Work of the Postpartum Doula

The role of a Postpartum Doula is like no other. A doula's role is fluid. From family to family, hour-to-hour, our role is constantly changing. In just one day, we may serve as educator, listening ear, puddle sitter, and source of encouragement. We offer practical support by preparing nutritious meals, nurturing older children, even going to the store for essentials. The doula recognizes when a family can benefit from specialized help and offers quality, reliable referrals when they are needed. At all times, the doula provides reassurance, support, and the belief that these parents can and will be successful in nurturing their family.

Another way to learn the role of the doula is to clarify what we do not do. We are not nursing specialists, therapists, or clinical care providers. Nor are we housekeepers or babysitters. While we do strive to help to keep the home organized and neat, we are not there to clean it. Similarly, while we engage with and nurture infants and their siblings, our role is not to replace the parents.

Doulas come alongside the family to provide them with the support that they need in real-time—as they need it. As parents and children move through stages of development and adjustment, our practical support and anticipatory guidance are available to them as needed.

There is a clear need for doulas to fill the overwhelming chasm many now find themselves in in the absence of traditional support. New families need not be left bereft. One family at a time, doulas educate and support. We create a community with our services, referrals to professionals, and peer support. We suggest or develop traditions to be assimilated by the families that we serve, and they can teach them to their friends, family, and eventually to their children. Providing the opportunity to recover from the birth experience can allow parents to gently move into new roles. Doulas make a difference in welcoming babies and their freshly evolved parents back into our society and helping them thrive.

Doula as a Generalist

Doulas—and those who are doula-ing new families—arrive during one of the most exciting and vulnerable experiences in life. Parents will come to trust you, sometimes in a profound way. This is why it is important to remain mindful of the sacredness of the relationship.

The doula can honor this trust by holding several concepts as priorities:

Remember that you are a *generalist*.

You know a great deal about many different things. Unless you are already trained as a specialist in a particular area, you are not an expert in anything but the norm. This means that your role is to screen and then know who to refer your clients to for help. Avoid overstepping boundaries and offering yourself as an expert when you are not. Make connections and really know what's available in your community. Strive to have a name and number to offer when expert advice is needed. Equally important is knowing where to look when you find that you yourself do not have the necessary information.

Respect everyone's right to parent in their own way.

You may be the only person to do this for them. Your personal priorities and philosophies can be applied to your own family. When doula-ing, support and encourage the parents in making their own decisions and developing their own style.

The doula role is fluid; whatever will best support the parents and nurture the new family is the primary task of the moment. The following are things that may happen on any given day as a doula. It is not an all-inclusive list, just a general idea of what many doulas do. What will you do as a postpartum doula? What will you not want to do?

Doulas often:

- ✓ Help parents to stay nourished and well hydrated.

- ✓ Facilitate nursing through positioning, snacks, and suggestions.

- ✓ Educate family members on the art of nurturing through modeling, demonstration, and explanation.

- ✓ Engage with older siblings.

- ✓ Nurture the baby while parents rest or play with older children.

- ✓ Help to insulate the family from a constant flow of communication and visitors (with their permission).

- ✓ Assist with bathing and dressing the baby or perform these tasks at the parents' request.

- ✓ Prepare meals.

- ✓ Organize for the next day by making sure that the diaper bag and changing areas are stocked.

- ✓ Set up *nests*. Assemble basics in a basket or bin for each commonly used area of the home. In addition to diapers, changes of clothes and receiving blankets, include basics for parents like snacks, a clean shirt, water bottles, phone chargers, and more.

- ✓ Sit and really listen as parents describe their day, feelings, and concerns.

- ✓ Listen to the birth story again and again.

✓ Make suggestions for resources, referrals, and networking with other parents.

✓ Answer questions.

✓ Assess skills and adjustment and make recommendations when appropriate.

✓ Answer the questions of other family members and visitors.

Doulas sometimes:

✓ Shop for groceries.

✓ Wash, fold, and put away the baby's and siblings' clothes.

✓ Offer a gentle and relaxing foot or shoulder rub.

✓ Run errands with or for the parents.

What on these list appeals? What sounds like you? What sounds not at all like you?

Our Role Is Consistent

Since our role places us directly in the lives of new families, there is the real possibility that just about anything can happen during that time. What might that look like? Expected challenges include baby blues, visiting family members creating stressful dynamics, and adjustment challenges in older siblings. Less common situations may include a death in the family, a parent for whom you are the sole support, an unforeseen disability or illness in the baby, severe anxiety or depression, or an abusive partner. Pretty much anything that can happen in life can happen during your time supporting a new family.

Some years ago, I sat down with Susan Martensen and Patricia Predmore, two experienced doula mentors, and we created an acronym to assist doulas through any possible eventuality: NEAR.

Nurture
Educate
Assess
Refer

At all times, a top priority is to *nurture* our clients, as well as any support people who may be present. We nurture with everything we do—with our calm presence, our listening without taking over, with food, guidance, full attention, and acceptance.

We are also almost always *educating*, not by pointing to a blackboard or book, but in more practical and subtle ways. When clients ask questions, we explain options available to them, with both their up- and downsides. When we wash our hands upon arrival, we are educating parents that hand washing is a priority. When we wear the baby in a carrier and prepare lunch while the parents nap or shower, we are offering them a strategy that they too can use to get through their day.

Every person is *assessing* at all times. It is so automatic that we don't even notice it. Where is the safest place to cross this street? That is an assessment. Does this person seem friendly and safe to talk to? Another assessment. Is there soap and a towel in the bathroom? Yet another assessment. These are the ways in which a doula is assessing. It is the act of noticing; doulas become expert at noticing. This is partially achieved by our lack of agenda. When a person arrives with an agenda, they are naturally going to hone in on observations specific to that agenda. The doula arrives with one top priority:

to support the family in the way that they need most at that moment. This allows us to absorb every situation and identify ways in which we can make a difference.

As doulas, we are also making *referrals* with some regularity. Sometimes these are to professionals who specialize in areas that are too specific to fall under our generalist umbrella: to lactation professionals, therapists, or health-care providers. Our referrals extend far beyond this, however. They include books and websites, resources for community and companionship, public programs—anything that can arise during the fourth trimester, therefore anything that can arise during life itself.

The doula can apply the NEAR acronym to any situation. Death in the family? Debilitating depression? Divorce? Medical complications? It's all the same. This proves helpful in a situation that is unfamiliar or overwhelming, where the path to appropriate support is not clear. Take some deep breaths, do way more listening than speaking, and then remember, "My role is to be NEAR." Your initial path will make itself clear.

Anticipatory Guidance

When describing doula support, *anticipatory guidance* is sometimes under-emphasized. The concept is that through our education and practical experiences, we have developed a heightened accuracy in what to expect next. The experience of parenting comes with its own developmental process, and the doula is a student of this process. While remaining mindful that each individual and family will develop in their own way, the doula's insights into typical newborn and family development will provide tools to help prepare for what may be coming next. This can facilitate smoother transitions.

Here is an example: Many babies are easier to care for in the first week or two. Parents often describe their babies as "really good," which commonly is a reference to their sleep patterns and degree of ease with which they can be soothed. If this is a first baby, it is possible to sleep when the baby sleeps. Older children may transition smoothly during these early days, since the baby is often asleep and requires minimal support with transitions.

At some point, often somewhere around the baby's third week, the new little person begins to wake up. This is a normal and healthy developmental change, yet it can wreak havoc. Whereas last week the baby could be fed, held for a few minutes, then put down to sleep, the baby in this new level of awakening may feed, doze off, then awaken and cry when laid down to sleep. Older children become frustrated when parents' time is spent on infant care and may feel that they are a lesser priority. Behavior escalates, and very quickly, a parent may feel overwhelmed.

How can anticipatory guidance help in this situation? Simply being aware of this common phenomenon can change everything. During an intake or prenatal visit, the doula can share this information with prospective clients and suggest that they extend their postpartum support to last through the first four to six—or longer—weeks for exactly this reason. (This doesn't necessarily mean upselling hours. The parent may choose fewer hours per week in order to extend the duration of doula support.)

Next, they remind the parents during those early weeks that this is a time for the family to recover from birth and adjust, and that things are soon going to change. Strategies such as babywearing to consistently meet babies' needs, and establishing rituals with older children, will go far in easing this transition.

The Mosaic of Postpartum Support

Imagine a mosaic of your choice, vibrant and dynamic in color. Now take this a step further and consider each of these colors to represent a different aspect of the support you provide as you doula a family. Perhaps light blue is listening. Green may represent the meals that you create. Dark blue is rest time for parents. Lavender is educating. Yellow is time spent with the children.

Postpartum doula mentor Susan Martensen created the mosaic of postpartum support to provide a framework for identifying the texture of a relationship with a family. She explains that when we are operating within our role, the mosaic will be colorful and dynamic. While some days and even weeks may be heavily colored by just a few hues, there should still be variation.

As time progresses and challenges diffuse, remaining colors offer insight as to potential ongoing needs of the family. If the role is colored heavily with childcare, the doula can help parents identify options for ongoing care. If the doula's focus is that of companion, connecting the parent with opportunities for meeting peers becomes our role. This invaluable tool rests quietly in our toolbox, available to keep both doula and client on the path of fostering independence.

Where Do You Come From?

What life experiences went into the creation of the current version of yourself? Do you know what it is about your history that has planted this desire to support others? Does your willingness to support stem from a seed of abundance? Are you seeking to pay forward the goodness you have received? Or are you perhaps growing after an experience of scarcity of support in your own life? Perhaps some of each? Neither is inherently good or bad; they are just what brought you to today. They are, however, worthy of consideration, because they will likely play into the way you perceive your role and possibly form expectations as you create relationships with the families you serve.

Your personal experiences of family shape your expectations of and reactions to the dynamics you encounter with your clients. Do you know what your buttons are? For example, you might feel a strong, almost primal reaction when parents smoke around their children. Raised voices might make you wince. Or you might be surprised when clients are quiet and reluctant to share when they are obviously disagreeing on a subject. Your founding relationships shape your expectations of caregiving and how best to go about it. Rather than trying to deny your own feelings, take the time to lean in and explore their origins and where they may be leading you.

You Will Not be Everyone's Match

I promise you will not be a match for everyone. Someone will find you too old, another too young. You have too much experience, too little, or your experience is in the wrong area. You will be overpriced, or your fees will be too low and therefore, suspicious.

You will be of the wrong political affiliation, skin color, or faith. Your tattoos will be off-putting, or you might not have enough tattoos. You will dress too conservatively or too casually. Your voice will sound just like Auntie Deborah, and they can't stand Auntie Deborah.

All this is to say, of course, that you won't be a match for everyone. It's impossible. It's also not personal. It will feel personal, and it can certainly feel hurtful, but their choice will have everything to do with themselves and nothing to do with you. We sometimes encourage potential clients to interview more than one doula in order to find their best possible match. Not every one of us uses this approach. Those who do, though, are engaging in an ongoing exercise in vulnerability—in the best possible way. A willingness to be compared to others shows that you are confident in what you have to offer. It also demonstrates that the birthing parents' comfort is your top priority.

Creating Acquaintance vs. Building Relationships

When we doula a family, we strive for more than to know them—our goal is to build lasting relationships. Knowing people is one-sided and is not necessarily linked with sharing and trust. Relationships are two-sided and include give and take. Relationships evolve. Relationships last. Relationships also require tending.

The process described below is a framework of information for getting to know a family and a potential launching point. The relationship itself will require ongoing attention, as do all relationships. Doulas bring a tenderness to our support not always seen in working relationships. The best way to provide a warm presence and hold space with people is to know and genuinely care about them.

How Do We Get There?

✓ Setting our intention of genuinely learning this family

✓ Communication

✓ Listening

✓ Allowing ourselves to be authentic and vulnerable

How Do I Get to Know My Clients?

Since you will be entering your clients' lives during a time of joy and also potential stress, it is ideal to get to know them as quickly as possible. Sometimes your relationship will begin while they are pregnant, and you can learn their wants, needs, and expectations in a relaxed setting during a prenatal visit. At other times, you will be hired after the birth, possibly even during a time of crisis such as a health or relationship challenge. In all situations, the goal is much more than getting to know your clients. The goal is to build relationships.

What Information Should I Cover During a Prenatal/Intake Visit?

The goal of this visit is to establish a working relationship with your clients, both in terms of support and administration. Objectives include:

✓ Ask each person, "What would you like me to know about you?"

✓ Ask, "What kind of support do you anticipate needing?" Pay close attention to the answer. If there is more than one family member present, ask them all.

✓ Ask about any cultural traditions that are a part of their family life.

✓ When applicable, provide information on nursing education and preparation.

✓ Help assess existing support networks and plan to fill gaps.

✓ Offer realistic expectations for the early postpartum weeks.

✓ Educate family members on the art of supporting the mother.

✓ Review basic coping skills for new parents.

✓ Explain what you have to offer them. Also explain any tasks that you do not perform or that are out of your scope of practice.

✓ Answer questions on common trends in parenting.

✓ Establish payment procedures.

✓ Establish an anticipated schedule for doula support.

✓ Supply contact information.

✓ Offer appropriate referrals.

✓ Determine if there are any medical conditions, food preferences, or allergies in the family that you should be aware of.

✓ Meet family pets.

Listen, Then Listen Some More

Many of us have come into contact with people during times of transition or conflict and are drawn to helping people during such times. The desire to help, to soothe, and to make things better is pure and generous. The manner in which this is accomplished can have a range of implications for both the family itself and the relationship between the doula and the parents. This is why it is so important for the doula to help parents to reach decisions and work through challenges independently. With support, but independently.

People need the opportunity to express their feelings: they need to feel that they have been heard. Once a person has expressed themselves, they can feel validated. Often during the process of describing a situation aloud, a person shares thoughts that lead them to discover a working solution.

Think of the common sitcom scenario when a character is speaking with a friend or parent, seeking advice. The person in crisis talks and talks, and the "helper" keeps trying to get a word in edge wise, with little exclamations like, "So . . ." and "B . . ." but keeps getting cut off by the speaker. At the end, the character seeking advice talks herself through to a solution. The scene ends with, "Thanks. I know what to do now. You give great advice."

This is what we are going for.

Doula Language

As doulas, we are responsible with our words. We don't leave them lying around for others to trip over after we've left. They are carefully considered and offered with respect and mindfulness. Doula language is open-ended, person-building, includes silence, and is fitted to the situation. We are aware that words matter. That people do not necessarily hear our good intentions. It's on us to make them stick.

Doulas might say:

✓ What does this mean to you?

✓ This must be hard.

✓ I wish I had words for this.

✓ I'm here, and we will do it together.

✓ My job is to support you in whatever you decide.

✓ It doesn't matter what I would do—you're the parents and will make the choices that are right for your family.

Client Language—Learn Theirs

One client stands out in teaching me the value of really listening to the words people use and the way in which they use them. My prenatal intake meeting at the home of this client felt relaxed and comfortable. She was enthusiastic in her pursuit of support and shaping her early parenting experience. I remember that her home felt so different from mine—still, quiet, thought out. It was lovely, she was lovely, and we were a great match doula-wise. She nodded and agreed with my description of my role. We agreed that I would come for a four-hour shift during the weekdays in her early weeks postpartum. She asked, ". . . and we'll have a meal together?" "If you'd like," I responded. On my ride home, I contemplated that exchange. On my end, I was grateful for the clarification of whether I'm expected to bring my own meal, or clients consider me a guest and want me to join them for meals.

In my early days, I felt awkward in having that conversation upfront. She had made it easy for me. I am a person of words; the words people choose and how they use them to stay with me; ". . . and we'll have a meal together?" There was something there. It was important, and I tucked that information away.

I remember this as being my only client in which the focus of my role felt like nurture through food. We did all the usual things: I observed and made recommendations on her breastfeeding, listened to her birth story, helped her to get naps, and connected her with a support community. In this case, though, the focus was on meals. While she napped, I would tuck her baby into my carrier and assemble lovely lunches for her. Since her home felt so thought out, I tried to create her meals the same way. Nothing fancy, but I sliced the avocado at pretty angles, and arranged the sandwich on the plate just so. We sat in her peaceful kitchen and chatted while we ate. After the first week or so, she asked me to get dinner started before I left, which I was happy to do.

After several weeks, she casually shared with me during lunch that she had an eating disorder. One aspect of that was that she was unable to eat alone. I realized that the meals and snacks we shared were the only food she was able to eat until another family member joined her, and her partner worked long hours. Everything clicked. I recognized that early on, when I was a stranger, this wasn't something she was comfortable sharing. Her open-ended suggestion was her only way of expressing her need. Fortunately, in this case, I was able to receive her subtle request and meet her needs. I am certain that hasn't always been the case, and that there have been other times when I've missed cues. Perhaps they weren't shared in a way that resonated with me. Perhaps I was tired, or my mind was cluttered, or I had too many tasks to complete during my visit to be an ideal listener. In this case, I succeeded.

This memory stays with me. It reminds me to put down my phone, not fiddle or busy myself with tasks at all times. Sometimes both speaker and receiver require stillness and focus to allow for genuine sharing. In a society where we value our ability to get things done, this can feel like an exercise in restraint, but given its worth, it is a practice worth cultivating.

Puddle Sitting

Doulas bring new families *presence*. At any time, and especially in times of challenge, our most powerful action may be inaction. Tidying and organizing and resourcing are all very helpful in times of need, but they are secondary offerings. First, we need someone to sit with us while we grieve, rage, or stare numbly at the walls. We need that person to be absent of agenda, to be comfortable with tears and silence, loud voices, and strong feelings. We need a puddle sitter.

Sheroke Ilse offers the following words of wisdom in her book, *Giving Care, Taking Care*: ". . . it is not your place to try to make it better. Rather, share your compassion and sit in their puddle, where they may need to wallow, complain, wail, cry, and show anger." Doulas are puddle sitters. We sit, listen, and wait in silence, signaling our acceptance of this person's experience. So simple. Simple, rare, and vital.

Thoughts on Advice—When Big Decisions are Being Made

This one is tricky because, as doulas, it really isn't up to us to give advice. The greatest gift we can offer parents is to encourage and respect their decision making. Honoring their intuition, priorities, and style will go further than any single other service we can provide; that doesn't make it easy, though. Significant life choices feel overwhelming, and it makes sense that parents may look to us for an answer. Keeping our advice to ourselves is *hard*. Probably way harder than you can imagine in advance. That's what makes it such a gift to new parents. If they could get that kind of support just anywhere, they wouldn't need us, would they?

What's challenging is that we've lived our own experiences, learned from them, and we just *know* what would make things so much better. Or, at least, we think it would improve things. Very likely, it would. Even then, not our role. We are planting seeds for a harvest that will take place way after our time in the field. We are fostering independence in people who will use the resulting sense of confidence throughout their parenting careers—standing up to family members, advocating for their children in school, and contending with medical decisions and challenging interactions that life may bring, to name a few. For these reasons, being just one of the countless people throughout their parenting experience to imply that they are unqualified in their role is counterproductive. Confident parents are the doula's goal, rather than creating any one style of parent.

As we doula parents, then, our role is to educate on options. Ideally, these options are evidence-based and researched rather than reaching into our emotional pockets for what feels comfortable and right to us. This allows us to grow as well, as we will sometimes observe a choice and result that we find surprisingly successful. We offer options, even when our clients specifically request our advice. "What would you do?" or "How did you handle this when your child was a baby?" feel like natural times to share our own experiences, but take a moment to consider whether your reply is a quick fix that keeps both parent and doula in their comfort zone or an opportunity to grow and stretch within roles. A simple, "My situation was different. What's your goal here? What would you most like to see happen?" can turn the focus back to the situation at hand and avoid a future sticky situation in which either you now bear emotional responsibility for the decision you encouraged, or your client feels uncomfortable because they made a different choice or were unable to do things your way.

Occasionally, you will share limited options or even an opinion, of course. One example that comes to mind on this would be something that has been overwhelmingly proven. For example, you may have clearly educated your clients on the need for frequent feeds when breastfeeding, or that newborns are not developmentally ready to sleep through the night in a room of their own. Your clients may have looked into your eyes, smiled and nodded, and made choices that were very different from your recommendations.

In these situations, open communication is key. Try offering your observation of behaviors rather than summarizing and labeling. In the example above, you might say, "I've noticed that you're working very hard to have India sleep in her crib through the night, but things are getting challenging. She's crying quite a bit, her weight has gone down, and you're expressing frustration when we talk." Make suggestions. In this case, you might offer resources on infant sleep. Offer to watch a video with them or to attend a new parent's group together to bring in another professional's opinion.

To summarize, the approach here is to offer our observations and make suggestions. If one approach isn't successful, try another way. While engaged in this challenge, remain mindful of your personal and professional boundaries. If you're feeling uncomfortable in either of these, remember that your experience is also important and valid. If parents make choices that leave you feeling unsafe in the care you're providing, it is acceptable to calmly voice this and offer to help them to identify a different professional better suited to their goals and strategies.

Challenging Conversations

Like it or not, there are times when difficult conversations become necessary. An obvious example of this would be when one or more parents are experiencing a challenging emotional adjustment. Another might be when a chosen strategy appears to be creating problems rather than solving them. Yet another could be when the doula feels that they are being asked to act outside of their role. In any of these circumstances, consider the following:

- ✓ Know that your perspective is valuable and valid.

- ✓ Remember that you are a generalist, rather than a specialist. Remember that your training is not specific, so your conversation should be general as well.

- ✓ Keep in mind that your observations and reactions are based on your own history, culture, education, and experiences in life and that others may see things differently.

- ✓ Cite specific observations without judgment and without adding your own conclusions.

- ✓ Stay within your role; do not diagnose (another form of judgment).

- ✓ Have a genuine open mind and strive to be open to seeing things differently.

- ✓ Avoid making generalizations and using labels.

- ✓ Keep calm. Develop skills in relaxing your voice and body so that you remain approachable.

Here's an example:

> Your client seems to spend a great deal of time crying during your visits. This, combined with other observations, have you concerned, and her partner seems to share that concern and has been reaching out to you with texts.

> You might suggest a team meeting and say,

> "Deborah, in my weeks here, I've noticed some things that I'd like to talk about. Sometimes when I arrive, I find you crying. Also, I've noticed that you don't seem to be honestly comfortable spending time alone with the baby. I'm wondering what your experience is of these observations?" We might later mention that there are things we know can help when people have had a baby: a social group of peers, sleep, eating well, staying hydrated, access to sunlight, and recovery-appropriate exercise. We can add, as appropriate, that at times, a therapist may have additional offerings that could help to lessen the challenges and allow for more enjoyment during this time of great change.

> Note the effort to avoid labeling, and that no judgment or diagnosis have been attributed to these behaviors outside of the initial request to talk. If there are additional family members, suggest including them in the conversation if the parents would find it helpful. Family members may themselves be struggling and could benefit from feeling heard in a constructive manner.

Another example:

> You have noticed that for your past several visits, the mosaic of support you are providing is now almost all one color, representing more of a childcare role than that of a doula. The first several times your client left the baby with you fell

under your role: first, she had a follow-up appointment with her midwife, and then a postpartum yoga class for the first time. Since then, she is mostly leaving upon your arrival, attending her yoga class, and meeting friends afterward. You recognize that this is no longer doula-ing and that your presence is providing a bandage rather than a long-term solution since, doubtless, she will have activities to attend throughout her parenting experience. You might say:

"Janei, in recent days I've noticed some things that I'd like to talk about. You are getting out and about now, and that's great! Taking care of yourself with yoga and spending time with friends are all exactly what you should be doing right now, and I'm happy that you felt safe leaving the baby with me as you tried those things out. Now that they're part of an established routine that's most of our doula-ing time, I'm thinking it's time for my role to change. Rather than being the childcare provider, my role is to help you to find one. That's what I'm seeing from where I am. What do you think?"

Again, rather than declaring your work done or adding any emotion or judgment to your part of the conversation, remaining open-ended allows space for your client to reply in whatever way they feel—which could be different from what you're expecting. They may share that they are, in fact, struggling with anxiety about leaving the baby, which opens up a new line of communication. We never know where someone is coming from until we ask them after making sure to create a safe space for sharing.

Family Dynamics

When we doula a family through their early parenting experience, we are present during a time both plump with joy and potential, and raw with the experiences of adaptation and vulnerability. It is a time of organic shifting of relationships. Daughter, son, partner, other—all dynamics in the family shift with the addition of a new person, transformation of the existing members, and redefining of roles.

In the midst of all the adaptation described above is the doula, or doula-ing person, who has the additional task of learning this family. What are we learning? How they work together. How they welcome and accommodate babies into their family. How they communicate support, as well as how they show disapproval. Where we can help, and where we need to stand back and honor that this is their family and things will unfold in their own way—which is not necessarily the way we would choose for them. Here is one of the most important things you can remember as a doula:

> **This is not your family. These are not your dynamics.**
> **The dynamics in place were there long before your arrival,**
> **and will likely remain long after you leave.**

This mantra is one that will benefit you more often than you can anticipate because, believe me, your clients' families do not work like yours. I can say this without knowing you or your clients because it is a universal truth. Even the families you meet that feel familiar may eventually surprise you by going in a different direction at some point.

Postpartum-support work is *life*. It can include perceived successes and failures, pain, relived trauma, power dynamics, feelings of self-worth, and crisis of self all wrapped in a tidy package that often includes sleep deprivation, physical recovery and changes, and financial stressors. People may make choices without the agreement of their partner (if they have one), with their support or seemingly to spite them. They may offer loving support in a manner you can't imagine experiencing. Or, just as easily, indifference you would find paralyzing.

As the caring observer immersed in the home, the doula suggests strategies gained through education and experience. It takes us by surprise, then, when they ignore our suggestions or go in the opposite direction.

These are the moments when doula support really happens. Honoring the choices of others when we disagree with them, when they've asked our opinion and then ignored it, and when a solution can seem so clear to us—this is true non-judgmental support. It means recognizing that we cannot expect others to make their life choices based upon *our* training and personal experiences. It means that while we may make a difference by introducing options and modeling caring support, we cannot change people or relationships. We are invited observers and helpers, and will make the greatest impact when we remain mindful of our roles.

Culture—Avoiding the Trap of "Everyone"

Whoever you are, wherever you are, you live within a particular culture. More accurately, you are a member of and interact regularly with any number of communities (Godin, 2008). One is your family: your family of origin as well as the family you may be raising. Another is your religious affiliation if you have one. You may have a parenting community, a school community, an art community, or an online community. Since this is who you interact with throughout your days, it's easy to feel as though your world is representative of the world at large. Let me take this moment to assure you that whatever you think everyone is doing, they aren't. While it may be accurate that many people within a particular age group, socioeconomic group, or geographic community are making common choices, that group is not everyone.

Let me explain; sometimes I hear doulas, especially successfully employed doulas, say things along the lines of, "Everyone is sleep training," or "Everyone uses video monitors." The more accurate statement is that many of their clients are making that choice. In such situations, I take the opportunity to point out that parents who are under-resourced and concerned about heat and safe housing are less likely to be using video monitors. I point this out not to make people feel uncomfortable but because language matters. Words are powerful. The words we use shape the way others think and also affect the way that we ourselves see things (Ruiz, 1997). When we use limiting language, we limit our expectations of others as well as our potential for growth.

The Significance of Culture

As a rule, humans cling to ritual. Historically, people have fallen back upon the rituals of their religious and ethnic communities during major events in their lives. When a couple meets and is ready to marry, they follow the traditions established by their culture. The courting process, ceremony, and even the clothing worn by the wedding party are dictated by the common practices of the community. Similarly, faced with death, people draw upon ritual to tell them how to behave and express their grief, as well as how to honor their family members. A third major event in the course of our lives is birth. The way that people bring their children into the world and welcome them reflects the experiences of their family and ancestors before them.

It is important for a new mother to feel safe and cared for in the weeks following her birth experience. Studies show that if a woman feels supported, she will have better success with breastfeeding, greater self-confidence, and is less likely to experience postpartum depression. Professionals working with birthing families must equip themselves with the skills needed to provide those families with the cultural sensitivity they deserve.

How Can We Support the Family's Traditions?

✓ Make no assumptions.

✓ Ask for a description of traditions.

✓ Offer to help with celebrations.

✓ Be sensitive to modesty preferences.

✓ Carefully observe and follow the examples of others.

✓ Be open about what you do and do not know.

✓ Respect differences non-judgmentally.

✓ Ask questions.

Challenges in Times of Transition—Experiences of Grief and Loss

As doulas, we are honored with the invitation to participate in the wonder and joy of new life every time we go to work. This means that we also experience the difficult realities that accompany any major life transition, and those that occur completely independent of one.

Grief can be experienced by anyone within the family dynamic, and it may not look or sound like the loss you anticipated in your doula work. In preparing to support families, our minds tend to turn toward obvious fears: illness or death of the newborn, prematurity, loss of a parent or grandparent, perhaps. These are universally relatable challenging outcomes, and we both dread and prepare for them (more on infant loss later in this book). What we cannot always be prepared for, and cannot always relate to, are those losses that are deeply personal to the individual. Losses that we may not identify with and therefore, may not have our eyes and ears open to. Loss of the pre-pregnancy body or pregnancy state are examples of this. The other-than-anticipated baby (looks, gender, differences) is another. Loss of focused interactions with a partner or older children also come into play: loss of spontaneity, or loss of a goal, career, project at work, or hobby. People hold many different things in their hearts and heads as priorities, and all such losses and grief are valid and deserving of acknowledgment and support.

In my own life as a doula, unique experiences of challenge opened me to inner struggles that might not be readily apparent. The elegant, slender-so-soon new mother who cut the covers off of magazines "so my husband won't look at them until I'm myself again." The mother with the thriving, robust new baby who regularly cried, grieving a baby who died at birth. The couple who missed their close pre-baby relationship to the point where they resented their baby. And so, so many more. Some may find a reflexive desire to encourage clients to focus on the positive, to compare or minimize. Better to listen, to accept the person for where and who they are and give them time to reconcile with their experience. It is possible to have more than one feeling at a time. It is also possible to honor all of them.

Be prepared to offer a safe place emotionally to anyone present during your visit. Remember that different people have different reactions: great sadness, anger, fear, or even what feels like an inadequate show of emotion are all normal. Individuals have varied coping skills and support needs. Keep your support open and honest. You can tell the parents that you wish you had the right words, but just don't know what to say. Tell them that you are there for them, in whatever way that they may need. Ask them for specific ways you can help or offer ideas of your own. Most importantly, validate their experience with listening and open-ended questions. Not everyone will make this space for them, but then again, not everyone is their doula.

A Note on Family Members with Differences

Babies born with disabilities or illnesses arrive with unknown potential, just like any other newborn. It can, however, be a difficult process for the parents who were not expecting this difference in their lives—and even when they were. They may experience a grieving process, as they've experienced a loss of a specific kind. The baby society raised them to expect, the "perfect" baby, is lost to them. Of course, there is no perfect baby, and there is no perfect person. All parents eventually learn their children's strengths and challenges. A difference here is that the initial discovery process is direct and intense. Parents in these situations do not have the luxury of easing into discovery. Their emotional adjustment, and sometimes daily lives, can reflect this. When children are born with differences, there is a steep learning curve on how to meet their needs, and parents are plunged into this experience fresh from the birthing room. Assessments, specialists, and treatments quickly become a part of everyday life from the very beginning.

This is another situation in which to remember your NEAR acronym: Nurture, Educate, Assess, and Refer. Distilled to its basics, the way to doula this family is exactly the same as any other situation. You may have had to do some quick learning about terminology and resources that are new to you, and that is just fine. Use this opportunity to model for parents that it's okay not to be automatic experts. Share when something is unfamiliar in a straightforward way, then explain your plan for networking, learning, and gathering resources and information.

Above all, remember that even when you don't know what to say, you can offer your heart and hands. Help the family in the way that they need. The best way to find out is to ask them and to really listen. Avoid supporting others in the way that you think they need, or the way that you would want to be helped yourself. Frequent check-ins are a must here, as you will all be learning this process together.

Parents as Informed Advocates

Life as a parent consists of seemingly benign bits of decision-making that, strung together, significantly impact the people our children are to become. The experience of building a life based on personal preferences and reflection rather than following along and reacting to what randomly flows our way is unusual in our culture. Consider this: were you taught or encouraged to deeply consider and act upon your knowledge and instincts? Are aspects of life that are actually choices generally accepted as a given?

Birth and early parenting plans are the first of a decades-long string of making choices about and for our children. School placement, navigating bullies, learning differences, and health challenges all require the gathering of information, making choices, and communicating those choices to others. What do parents need in order to advocate for themselves and their families? Successful advocacy requires:

✓ Confidence

✓ Access to accurate information

✓ Options

✓ Skill in relating to others

With the fostering of independence as a top objective, doulas can strive to remain mindful of ways to help our clients develop these skills. We help parents build confidence by believing in them and demonstrating that belief regularly. This means encouraging parents to check their own instincts on the needs of their children, rather than deferring to us, family members, or generalized policies found online. Take every opportunity to praise successes. Lead by following, rather than feeding your own confidence and feeling the expert. Stepping into the role as an advocate of the parents is hard, as it involves vulnerability—vital to success, but something that many of us do our best to avoid (Brown, 2015). Early moments like choosing where and when a baby sleeps, feeding approaches, and soothing strategies will eventually grow into confidence in meeting their child's needs. Fostered, this translates into parents who can advocate for educational, health, and social needs as the child continues to grow.

Accessing and vetting information is a life skill that not everyone possesses. Take time to consider what you know about researching. Do you know how to tease evidence-based information apart from online chatter? Do you understand that there are times when very official-seeming information is actually the marketing tool of a powerful industry? Learning to differentiate is a skill that requires ongoing effort. A good start for the doula is to read about how to understand the basics of research (Greenhalgh, 2014), as well as which early parenting clearinghouse websites are reliable, such as Choices In Childbirth. It's easier for you as the doula to offer parents insight into the process of information-gathering when you have some experience with it yourself.

Once we know how to investigate, we have options, even when the experts don't mention that we do. Second opinions, networking, consultations, and research all foster options.

Skill in relating to others is what brings it all together. Listening respectfully goes far in a successful negotiation, and so does expressing confidence in one's own knowledge and the expectation of being treated well in return. Remaining friendly and non-threatening can be challenging in the emotionally heated moments of parenting choices. Model these behaviors in any experiences of this nature in the early months. For example, avoiding or resolving a clash related to breastfeeding with a pediatrician or family member can extend into improved interactions in the future.

A Note on Advocacy

As a person who is drawn to doula work, you may already see your role as one of advocacy, whether for your own family or those you support. Experience has shown me that not everyone feels empowered or even positive about the things that excite me. I remember an intake phone call with a woman expecting twins. It was early in her pregnancy, and I enthusiastically shared with her what I know about nutrition and multiples pregnancy. I told her about my own twins, who were each over six pounds, twins who were born at over seven pounds each, and even clients whose babies' combined weights were exactly seventeen pounds.

She was quiet, and I erroneously assumed that she was dazzled by this information. I couldn't have been more wrong. She took a breath and laid into me; "How dare you imply that I have any control over whether these babies are born prematurely?! That is just awful!" I quickly understood that she took my words as proactive victim-blaming, which certainly wasn't my intent. My goal was for her to feel some degree of control and competency within her body, which can be difficult to maintain in highly medicalized multiples pregnancies. I did not meet my goal. We chatted awkwardly for another moment or two, then said goodbye. Obviously, she didn't hire me; I hope I didn't turn her off of doulas altogether.

While we have very different perspectives, I see this woman as one of my life-teachers. She reminded me that each person has their own innate personality and is shaped by their life experiences. To me, the thought of taking control of my pregnancy and birth is inspiring, while for others, it can be threatening and overwhelming. I hold this knowledge close in my support role. It helps me remember that both goals and the path for attaining them only succeed when they are set by the person themselves. It also helps me to remain still and patient inside when a path feels clear to me, and my clients seem unwilling to take it. I remember this doula error of mine and wish this mother well whenever I live the lesson she taught me.

Nurturing the Entire Family

Families are singular organisms composed of any number of interrelated individuals. All are connected. Most of us live or have lived as part of families. If one individual is unhappy or unwell, all are affected. When tension exists between two or more people, it pulls the entire entity out of shape. For these reasons, if doula support focuses solely on mothers and babies, it is akin to a medical professional treating a single body part rather than the whole person.

Doula trainings offer space for sharing, and over the years, I've been struck by how many see their roles as solely mother/baby support. One subset of attendees voices that they are "in it for the babies." They adore babies and love to hold them and care for them. Another subset arrives planning to "empower women." This is interesting to me because, from my perspective, the only person who can empower someone is that same person—themselves. Regardless of what brings you to this role—mothers, babies, other—if you're not supporting the family as a complete entity, you're potentially doing harm, or at the very least, not helping as much as you could. Ignoring one family member negates the wholeness of the unit. The doula who spends all their time with the baby is not contributing to the early bonding experiences that shape parent/child relationships. The doula who avoids fathers is not only depriving that person of support; they are also depriving the children of a potentially more confident and invested parent, and the mother of a partner who is educated on the art of support.

Doulas are people too, and our personal preferences are inherent. I ask you to engage in introspection and identify any strong feelings about who you do and do not feel comfortable supporting. Ask yourself questions; explore, and put your doula-ing and resourcing skills to work for yourself, if appropriate. Next, identify what you need to feel safe and comfortable as you doula a family. How can you build a role for yourself that is inclusive of family members while respecting your own needs for comfort and safety? Again, this is a moment that requires individuation and balance, and I do not have the answers. I include this section because in my own experience, simply being mindful of a challenge impacts my own behavior. Perhaps it works this way for you as well.

Defining Boundaries

What do you think of when you consider the word boundary? While it is woven into all of our interactions, both physical and emotional, how often do you consider it, or even why you should?

When doula-ing a family, boundaries work in both directions—they protect us, and they protect the families we serve.

Boundaries are the space between competing experiences. They include:

✓ The space between something that makes you feel comfortable and uncomfortable.

✓ The space between actions that are beneficial to you and those that aren't.

✓ The space between actions that are beneficial to your clients and those that aren't.

✓ The space between where "you" end and "I" begin (Katherine, 1994).

✓ The space between where you feel respected and disrespected.

✓ The space between privacy and exposure.

✓ The space between safe and unsafe.

✓ The space between your role and outside of your role.

All of us have lived with boundaries—their cushioning as well as their absence, and have been shaped by our experiences. Some people react strongly, building boundaries around every experience they meet. Others find themselves feeling adrift, unable to articulate their boundaries. This can leave them feeling vulnerable and taken advantage of. Most people move in and out of comfort around identifying and expressing their boundaries. When possible, identify yours ahead of time and use proactive and positive methods to communicate them. Carefully considered contracts and policies fall in this category. Just as important is frank, open conversation.

Living our boundaries and feeling comfortable with expressing them are among the best strategies for their successful maintenance. Communicating these can be straightforward and still kind; "Actually, that's not in my role/comfort zone, but resourcing is. Let me help you to find what you're looking for."

Life keeps bringing new experiences, and at times, we are unaware that a personal boundary exists until we seemingly walk right into it. We cannot anticipate every situation. When something feels "just wrong," take the time and emotional space to consider where that feeling is coming from. Once you've identified the breach, problem-solve around it. What needs to change? How can you best communicate that need? How can you facilitate it? It falls upon each of us to maintain the boundaries we need to feel safe and effective in our role. This life skill requires ever-evolving tending and introspection. Stick with it. You're worth it.

Other Voices on the
Art of Support

Sensitivity: The Source of a Doula's Magic

by Amy Gilliland

Most of what doulas do is based on interaction. Think about it. Our primary activities are communicating, connecting, and relating to other people. The care we offer is relationship-based, whether we've known the family for several months or a few hours. It's based on caring for them as individuals and using our knowledge to serve them in having the best experience possible. Building a rapport is based on reading cues correctly and responding appropriately. People feel that their doula "really got me" whenever sensitivity skills are effective. Cultivating sensitivity can bring you increased satisfaction with your own work and relationships, as well as increase your client's enjoyment with having you as their doula. No one else emphasizes meeting emotional needs as much as doulas do during the perinatal period.

Postpartum doulas rely on their sensitivity skills. They help you to read babies and parents, think more creatively to solve problems, and increase your communication effectiveness in talking and listening. When you're a sensitive communicator, other people often feel cared for, tended to, and understood. They feel safer with you and have fewer stress hormones.

As a long-time birth doula, trainer, and researcher, I've pondered what makes some birth and postpartum doulas successful and why others flounder. It isn't a lack of commitment or desire to be effective. It isn't a lack of business savvy. To me, the most critical doula skill is **sensitivity**; the ability to read another person's cues accurately and respond appropriately in a timely manner. Sensitivity is a primary component of emotional intelligence and a key skill in successful parenting and creating secure attachment in infancy. (This is different than an attachment parenting style.)

Over and over again, I see this critical skill making a major difference in their client and personal relationships. So many research participants told me that their doula seemed to read their minds by knowing what they needed without the person having to ask for it. They also described their doula's ability to understand what they were feeling without the need for words as "magical." But for doulas, it is the essential skill of reading people and interpreting their behavior accurately. It's using our brains, not magic. The good news is that we have the innate ability to learn and improve this skill; our brains are pre-programmed for it.

Most of what doulas do is based on interaction. Think about it. Our primary activities are communicating, connecting, and relating to other people. The care we offer is relationship-based, whether we've known the family for several months or a few hours. It's based on caring for them as individuals and using our knowledge to serve them in having the best experience possible. Building a rapport is based on reading cues correctly and responding appropriately.

Let's break down sensitivity into three steps, using parents and infants as an example. First, mothers and fathers need to learn to read their baby – to figure out from the baby's communications what the baby needs. Two, they need to respond in a way that answers the baby's needs. Third, they need to respond in a timely and contingent manner, so the infant knows that the parent's actions are in response to his or her communication behavior. Some common infant communication behaviors are smiling and eye contact, indicating a desire for social interaction; looking away, fussiness, indicating hunger, desire to be left alone, messy diaper, crying, indicating a need for soothing and assistance in regulating difficult emotions, overstimulation, etc.

Some babies are harder to read than others, so sensitivity also means trying different strategies and keeping at it until something works to help this particular baby. Children learn emotional regulation from sensitive parenting. Infants learn over time to deescalate their own internal states through the parents' soothing response to their child's intense emotions. As humans, we learn sensitivity by being responded to in a sensitive manner and being taught how to do so.

In a doula context, the most important aspect of sensitivity is the ability to read behavioral cues. We need to be able to read parents and figure out what their behaviors mean. We also need to read partners, grandmothers, and other care providers. If we break down the skill of reading others, the first action is *noticing*. We have to be paying attention to others and notice their cues. Something a person does enters our awareness. Second, we decide whether that behavior is worth paying attention to. For example, pushing glasses on the nose usually has little emotional meaning. Over time, effective readers usually develop accurate mental lists of what is worthy of attention.

Third, doulas need to generate different interpretations of the observed person's behavior. Our minds make a list of what it could mean. We look for more evidence that supports any of the possibilities we've thought of. Four, we settle on a likely interpretation and continue to monitor for more information. Research suggests that effective readers don't assume behavioral meanings but think of different possibilities for why people act in certain ways. They are also more aware of subtle cues, not just overtones. The truth is, your body is always communicating. Our nonverbal behavior is constantly revealing our internal state to others; it's called *nonverbal leakage*.

Most cues from adults are subtle, and some are idiosyncratic. For example, crossing the arms is generally thought to be a defensive posture. However, it also relieves tension in the shoulder muscles, so someone might not be defensive at all but have shoulder tension. When signals seem contradictory or ambiguous, you need to seek more information, even asking, to read this individual better.

After reading cues, doulas then need to act. We choose our own response based on our interpretations. Our responses need to be appropriate to the situation and the person, done in an appropriate time frame, and be connected to the behavior we've observed (contingency).

We can also share our observations with parents; "I notice that when you look your baby in the eyes, you give a deep sigh. Did you realize that? I was wondering what if it means anything to you."

Debriefing the Birth

Discussing the birth with the person who labored can have significant consequences. It is never a casual conversation, even though the setting might seem casual. As a doula, you don't know how the person feels about what happened, and you don't want to assume. You want to withhold judgment and pay attention to the speaker's behavioral cues. There are often a lot of verbal and nonverbal mixed messages. For example, the words might be, "I was fine when we went ahead with the Pitocin." But the nonverbal leakage might indicate tension (folded arms, stiff shoulders, eye gazing to the one side of the room).

In a counseling situation like this, you aren't expected to be a mind reader. You often need to ask about their feelings when observing these conflicting messages. This is a prime time to use your sensitivity skills and to confirm that what you perceive is actually accurate. "Even though you said you were okay with the Pitocin, I noticed that your back was stiff and arms were tense. What else are you thinking or feeling about that time?"

Remember that the person who is speaking about this intense experience is figuring out what it means as they talk. As the words reach the air, the speaker may be surprised by what they are saying or feeling as they recall their memories. Our role as sensitive observers is to be a mirror; gently pointing out what we notice about that person's behavior that may be below their level of awareness. In those first few conversations, people are often surprised by their conflicting emotions.

As doulas, we often fight our own urges to fix things or make them better. We don't want people to feel icky; we want to change that. But in this context, that gets in the way of the person reaching their own revelations or "aha" moments. Our role is to be present with their strong emotions, without trying to fix them or make them be any different than what they are. We are just present with them, without leaving, helping them to understand their own feelings better. The only way out of these strong emotions is by expressing them fully with another person who isn't scared of them. That can be us if we are sensitive to this process.

Conclusion

Paying attention to a parent's cues and responding appropriately to those cues could mean the difference between a painful experience or a peaceful evening. Although these sensitivity skills were acquired in an arduous way, they can be used very effectively as an adult.

Learning Exercises for Increasing Your Sensitivity Skills

The four steps of sensitivity provide different areas for skill development. You may be very strong in one area and weak in another. The good news is that daily life provides many opportunities for increasing one's sensitivity skills.

✓ Noticing

When you are alone, spend some time in a public place where there are different groups of people socializing (e.g., mall food court). Choose a person you can watch unobtrusively. How are they standing? What are the expressions on their face? Does it change when they are talking to someone else? Is there a lot of variety in their body posture or facial expression? As you are noticing them, also notice your own responses to this person. Are you interpreting their behaviors to mean something? What makes you think your assigned meaning is the correct one? For now, suppress your desire to think you know what they are feeling. Just pay attention to noticing this person's subtle and overt nonverbal communication signals. Even something as simple as a nose swipe with a finger may mean something. The objective here is to pay attention and see how much communication is occurring below this person's level of awareness. Go through this exercise, observing three different people. If one of them isn't working out (i.e., focusing on their smartphone), choose someone else. Stop before your brain gets tired; you want to "turn on" your noticing neurons but not fatigue them.

✓ Worthy of Attention

Of the behaviors you witnessed, which ones seemed to be communicating an internal state or important thought? Watch someone in a conversation now. Make a mental list of their "nonverbal leakage" (scratching ear, grimace, smile, looks away, looks down, looks at speaker). Which of those actions reveal something? Was the grimace in response to his ear or what the speaker said? Training yourself to discern what is important and what isn't usually takes feedback and the involvement of a trusted person. One of the reasons many of us have communication breakdowns is because we don't pay attention to the correct signals, or we interpret what those signals mean incorrectly.

For this exercise, spend time with a person you trust who is willing to help you. Tell them you are going to pay attention to their signals and repeatedly ask what they mean. Choose a simple activity where you are both doing something and talking but not so involved that you can't stop and discuss what you notice (playing a game, baking cookies, moving furniture, etc.). Suppress your tendency to "know" what that behavior means; instead, be genuinely curious. You may find that they are puzzled by their own behaviors, become irritated, enjoy the exercise, or start doing the same thing to you. This exercise can often be enlightening. I urge you to repeat it with several people to increase your awareness.

✓ Assigning Meaning

Hopefully, by doing the second exercise, you noticed how you automatically tend to interpret people's behaviors. Human beings naturally assign meaning; it is a survival skill designed to help us discern a potential threat. The problem is that once we assign a meaning, we often have an emotional response to that assigned meaning. It's that emotional response that gets us into trouble. For example, road rage is an emotional response based upon an interpretation of someone else's driving behavior. I have had to drive with a screaming baby, taking people in pain to the emergency room, and on the days each of my parents died. So, one of my main interpretations of other driver's behavior is "they may not be at their best" and as a result, are driving poorly.

This exercise is designed to heighten your awareness of your tendency to assign meaning. Go back to the mall, farmer's market, or other public place to observe people. Choose a group and observe one or two people in the group. Notice what each of your two people are doing and make up all the possible reasons they might be doing that behavior. If a person is shifting their weight from one foot to another, they might be impatient, bored by the person who is speaking, have shoes that are too tight, need to finish their errands, want to text but know that would be rude, or have to pee. Brainstorm a list of all the possibilities to the point of absurdity. Do this repeatedly until you free yourself of the tendency to "know" exactly why a person does anything. You want to engage your imagination in the art of interpretation.

✓ Interpreting Correctly and Choosing a Response

Once again, choose a person you know intimately and do something together, explaining that this time, you will tell them what you notice *and* what you think it means. *Be aware of your own tendency to have an emotional response to the meaning you have chosen.* As much as you can, set aside your emotional response. This exercise is about your self-awareness and tendency to interpret things in a certain way. The benefit of doing it with a friend is that you get to check the accuracy of your interpretations. So, choose someone who isn't easily miffed.

I would recommend doing this exercise with several different people. After doing it once or twice, make it a mutual exchange. It can be very enlightening to see how other people interpret *your* behavior and how those interpretations may affect your relationship. As an example, in my household growing up, the louder you closed a cabinet or a door, the angrier you were. This was a subtle signal of emotional distress. Whenever my husband slams a cabinet shut, I immediately think, "What's wrong?" Because of a childhood of conditioning, I have to calm down my inner alert system. But the first step is awareness that I've been conditioned to feel a certain way. I can't make it go away, and I can't stop my husband from doing it; he grew up with ten kids, so no one ever noticed a slamming door.

The next step in this exercise is to ask, "What do you want me to do when you act that way?" There are some basic possibilities: ignore it, address it directly, or address it indirectly. One's responses can be verbal, nonverbal, or a combination. In the cabinet example, my husband and I worked it out that the first response is I am supposed to ignore it. If my coping responses are very low that day, then I get to ask him to alter his behavior. He doesn't want to make me feel worse, but he doesn't want to change something that really is *my* problem.

Conclusion:

I have noticed that doulas who have had experiences where paying attention to others was critical for their survival or well being tend to have very effective sensitivity skills. Paying attention to a parent's cues and responding appropriately to those cues could mean the difference between a painful experience or a peaceful evening. Although these sensitivity skills were acquired in an arduous way, they can be used very effectively as an adult.

Cultivating sensitivity can bring you increased satisfaction with your own work and relationships; as well as increase your client's enjoyment with having you as their doula. No one else emphasizes meeting emotional needs as much as doulas do during the perinatal period. We know how important they are to a person's well being and sense of self worth, and the research backs us up. Sensitivity is the magical aspect of our skill set; when we know what someone needs before they do. It makes a difference in daily life care activities, and in formal debriefing conversations. We are present during intense life transformation in our client's lives; using your enhanced sensitivity skills can help things progress more smoothly.

References:

Benzies, K.M. & Magill-Evans, J. (2015) Through the Eyes of a New Dad: Experiences of First-Time Fathers of Late-Preterm Infants. *Infant Mental Health Journal*, 36(1), 78-87.

Biringen, Z., Derscheid, D., Vliegen, N., Closson, L. & Easterbrooks, M.A. (2014) Emotional availability (EA): Theoretical background, empirical research using the EA Scales, and clinical applications. *Developmental Review*, 34(2), 114-167.

Bryan, A.A. (2000) Enhancing parent-child interaction with a prenatal couple intervention. MCN: *The American Journal of Maternal/Child Nursing*, 25(3), p. 139-45.

Jonas, W., Atkinson, L., Steiner, M., Meaney, M.J., Wazana, A. & Fleming, A.S. (2015) Breastfeeding and maternal sensitivity predict early infant temperament. *Acta Paediatrica*, 104(7), 678-686.

Kivijarvi, M., Voeten, M., Niemela, P., Raiha, H., Lertola, K. & Piha, J. (2001) Maternal sensitivity behavior and infant behavior in early interaction. *Infant mental health journal*, 22(6), 627-640.

Mastergeorge, A.M., Paschall, K., Loeb, S.R. & Dixon, A. (2014) The Still-Face Paradigm and bidirectionality. Associations with maternal sensitivity, self-esteem and infant emotional reactivity. *Infant Behavior & Development*, 37(3), 387-397.

McMurtry, C.M. (2014) How do I love thee? Let me count the ways of responding and regulating. *Pain*, 155(8), 1421-1422.

Shin, H., Park, Y.J. & Kim, M.J. (2006) Predictors of maternal sensitivity during the early postpartum period. *Journal of Advanced Nursing*, 55(4), 425-434.

Stern, D. (1985) *The interpersonal world of the infant: a view from psychoanalysis and developmental psychology*, Basic Books, New York.

Supporting New Families as a Professional Doula

Try Another Way

If one thing doesn't work (for your doula practice or for your clients), try another way.

I wish I could cite which college professor taught me this life-enhancing message, but I did take the opportunity to research the concept, and sure enough, it's published in a special ed training manual (Gold, 1980), which makes sense, since that was my area of study. I will share with you the essence of the message, the mantra that I have extended to my doula work.

While working with families, be prepared to try numerous strategies before finding one that works. This applies to any aspect of your experience with them, but here are some areas:

✓ Nursing positioning

✓ How to communicate with a particular family member

✓ How you can best support a particular situation

✓ Teaching a skill

If one thing doesn't work, try another way. The options are truly unlimited. With your doula practice, the same applies:

✓ In creating your contract and other materials

✓ In marketing yourself

✓ In finding your doula community

✓ In identifying your skills and matching them with the corresponding client population

The concept of instant success is inaccurate. Successful business owners, artists, and relationships don't just pop up. Invest the time, the thought, and the forgiveness in yourself and others to be flexible. To fail. To persevere. To try another way.

Confidentiality

Ours is a sacred role. We have been invited to share time with a family during one of the most permeable and potentially fragile moments in their lives. Respect is foremost in active, conscious support of families. Above all, respect their privacy. Do not discuss your clients with friends, peers, or other professionals. If you do need to ask advice from someone else, the advice should be about your own role. Do not discuss your clients using names, private information, or any identifying information, to include where they live, age/gender of children, or birth outcomes.

Any information of theirs that you keep in written form needs to be locked—a locking file cabinet or a password to enter files on your computer. Also, consider the transfer of records when you are traveling to and from people's homes—what can you do to ensure that their information is secure, with no chance of accidentally dropping someone's personal information while in transit?

Once you've developed your approach regarding confidentiality, share it with your clients. Share it during your intake visit. Done right, it will impress them with your professionalism. Continue to share your confidentiality practices during your time working with the family. They are trusting you with not only their baby but also the intimacies of their family life together. The more secure they feel, the more they can open themselves to vulnerability and relax into their new role.

More on Confidentiality

In the U.S. today, many of us are living our lives as intimate strangers, with a majority of connectedness being lived online. Instagram, Twitter, Facebook—we know intimacies of people even tangentially involved in our lives. We watch their children grow up, learn of their sorrows and political views, all without interacting in real life, looking in their eyes, or hearing their voices.

This particular connectedness comes with its benefits and downsides. It means that someone can always be there, day or night. It means that we have access to nearly endless resources. It also means that we are only seeing people's chosen best sides, sometimes considering ourselves inferior because our lives don't match everyone else's constructed portfolio. As parents, it can mean opening ourselves to the inspection and criticism of large numbers of people, many of whom would never be privy to such intimacies before we lived our lives online. Those people can be insensitive or even cruel.

It also means that we have, as a society, set a baseline of comfort with sharing intimacies. In today's world, many people don't think twice before sharing photos, experiences, and feelings. As a support person involved in the lives of new parents, we will experience many feelings around their stories, and may even feel that the stories are our own, because we are a part of them.

They are not our stories to tell.

If we were there with them for the event, it's not our story to tell.

If we have strong feelings and need to process, it's not our story to tell.

If we are amazed and delighted and want to shout to the rooftops about how wonderful they are, it's not our story to tell.

If we find an image striking and touching, it's not our story to tell.

Take the time to carefully construct your policies around social media and review them thoroughly with your clients, and then review them again, after the baby is born. Before posting anything that is not your story, question your own motivation. Consider the code of ethics of any organization you are certified through. Consider your own morals. Most importantly, engage in conversation with the new parents.

On Dazzling Your Clients: It's More Complex Than You May Think

Early on in my doula career, a subconscious goal of mine was to impress my clients with my competency. I call it a subconscious goal because I didn't know it was there until I noticed the impact it was having on our relationships. Here's what I mean:

I am a mother of twins, and as a result of that, I'm frequently hired by families expecting multiples. My own parenting experience combined with the ongoing flow of multiples to practice with have really honed my skills; I can safely feed, burp, or transfer two babies while making it look easy, which it is not. My clients watched me perform and would sometimes let out a great sigh and observe, "I don't know if I'll ever be able to do things as well as you." "Of course, you will!" I'd chirp. "It comes with time and experience!"

Here's the thing, though. The more families I supported, the more I noticed that I was wrong. Not all people have the physical or emotional dexterity required to safely maneuver multiples with a smooth flow. Some people spend their parenting experience carrying or nursing their babies one at a time, and my behavior was leading to feelings of inadequacy. I was blocking my own goal of helping them to find their way and celebrate their own style and successes. It was a challenging internal moment.

With time, I backed off of my uber-competency. I slowed down and developed a style that was more considered and focused on modeling. I started to problem solve aloud to the babies; "Hmmm... How to get both of you and all of our supplies to the bath safely? Let's see..." I don't remember clients being dazzled by my physical prowess after those early years of doula-ing. I consider that to be a sign of my personal growth.

The Team Meeting

The team meeting can be a powerful tool in your doula bag. Its value lies in its versatility—it can be used for minor tweaking or in significant life situations. With a little set-up work in advance, the team meeting will take you far.

The concept is this: during your intake visit, explain to your clients that you require a weekly check-in team meeting. The team would be comprised of the doula(s), parent(s), and any other close family member or friend who is involved in the ongoing support of this family, such as a grandparent. It can take place in person, by phone, or virtually. The idea is to provide check-ins so you can be sure you're on track with the support you are offering and make recommendations as the situation evolves. It is usually brief and includes goal-setting for the upcoming days of service.

With many clients, this may be all the team visit ever needs to be. In times of challenge, it presents naturally as an already established venue for communication. The team meeting could be used when you are feeling concerned about a family member's emotional or physical recovery journey. It could be used to discuss the mosaic of support you are providing and any recommendations for how to enhance it. It could also be used to communicate personal or professional boundary breaches. Regardless of the reason, the approach is the same: share your observations, listen more than you speak, offer recommendations, and remember that you are a valid and worthy member of the team.

Working Together: The Importance of Back-Up

There are options in how to conduct your doula practice, and each comes with benefits and drawbacks. Begin by considering your own needs and how flexible you are in terms of working hours and wages earned. The goal is to find a match between what you have to offer and what is available to you. Remember that you can always change your approach. Choices available include:

✓ Working Independently

You can set your own hours, the income is all yours, and you run the show. You also assume all marketing and financial obligations, which may or may not play to your strengths. As a solo practice, you may be limiting the families that you're able to take on since they would be limited by your own availability. You'd want to be sure to have backup in case of emergency or overlapping clients. It's important to note that backup means different things to different doulas. Backup in some situations is a loose, verbal agreement. More of a "Will you be around in June? I have a client due and need someone, just in case." To other doulas, backup arrangements are more structured, with written agreements, payments for reserving time on call, and the backup doula meeting the parents. After you've given this thought, and have created your own vision, share it while building your doula relationships. Clear communication as you form back-up arrangements is to everyone's benefit.

✓ Working for an Agency

Typically, the business owner or manager takes care of the marketing and administration. They also perform the task of filling gaps if the doula calls in sick or has overlapping clients. All you have to do is provide excellent care. The cost of this diminished responsibility is that you will probably make significantly less money and have less overall autonomy.

✓ Doula Partnerships and Cooperatives

Very effective when you build a like-minded group of doulas who are willing to share clients and shifts, as well as responsibilities. Beneficial for all with less expense. It does take work to find that group of people who work well together and keep communication going, and tending those relationships is an ongoing process. Back up arrangements and payment arrangements will vary.

✓ Starting your Own Agency

Again, there are real benefits. With time, you may do better financially. You may be able to focus on administrative tasks and work with clients less often if your personal life isn't flexible at present. This is appealing for some. On the downside, you are in charge and can expect all of the challenges that come with the title.

Once you've decided on a strategy, the next step is to go out and find the amount of work that you are looking for. In the early years and perhaps for longer, you should expect to spend as much time on marketing and administration as you do actually working with clients. Make no mistake; you are, in fact, a business. Marketing is addressed later in this book.

What Kind of Hours Will I Work as a Postpartum Doula?

Many new doulas come into the field of doula support with families, often with children still living at home. Others have another career in place, which they are hoping to balance. The average doula, then, is not available to work 24 hours a day, and not necessarily even five days a week, and that is just fine.

Support needs differ for every family. Some need almost constant care, and there's no way you can provide all of it. This is where networking with other doulas is helpful. If you have a potential client, you can join with another doula, working the hours you have available and satisfying the needs of the client at the same time. Be upfront and tell potential clients when you are realistically available. Sometimes you will be a match, other times not. Families are often willing to work around the schedule of a doula who they feel a strong connection to.

When my children were school-aged, the majority of my doula work took place during the hours of 10 am and 3 pm. This allowed me to wave as my children boarded the bus and again when they arrived home in the afternoon. When time allowed, or our bank account required it, I made myself available to work additional shifts. Some clients were on my own, while others were shared. That flexibility allowed me to draw a genuine living income that fit the needs of my family. There were times when I felt like I worked almost constantly, and others when family life got tough and I could hardly work at all. One reassuring aspect of doula work; people will always be having babies. If life requires you to take a break for a bit, you can come back when you're ready, and the new families will still be there.

What are Common Shifts Worked by Postpartum Doulas?

Some doulas are set in their shifts, with policies such as, "We work from 9 to 5 every day." The benefits here are that scheduling is easier, the pay is higher due to working more hours, and the doula loses less time in commuting for shorter shifts. One risk is that clients may be put off emotionally or financially by a lack of options. Additionally, it may be more hours of support than they require. Interestingly, an overabundance of downtime can lead to boundary transgressions in doula support. In other words, the doula may perform tasks outside of the role as a way of substantiating their presence.

Other doulas prefer to offer more flexible, shorter shifts. Parents benefit from knowing that someone will be there at some point, and do not need continuous care. The knowledge that there will be an opportunity for a shower, nap, or grocery shopping helps to relieve stress. Benefits here include that the doula can maintain another job (doula or other work), and more easily meet responsibilities at home. The risk is potentially less income: fewer hours worked for the same commuting time.

Common shifts worked by doulas include:

Days

Either a standard 9 to 5 shift, or a short, flexible 3 to 5-hour shift, such as 10 am to 2 pm.

After School

Say, 2 to 5 or 6 pm.

Evenings

About 6 pm until "bedtime," around 10 or 11 pm.

Overnights

Perhaps from 9 or 10 pm through an agreed time in the morning. During this time, rather than replacing the parent, we continue the role of active support during the night. Parents welcome a calming, supportive presence during feeding, someone to fill the water glass, make a snack, and change diapers. Questions arise, and babies require care just as often as they do during the day. This is especially helpful for parents with multiples.

Over the years, I've worked many overnights. Often, those were families going through the challenges of babies not yet nursing, so nights involved a constant cycle of pumping, feeding the baby expressed milk or formula, cleaning pump supplies, and helping parents get some rest. I've supported mothers who had been hospitalized for postpartum depression, and part of their prescription for recovery was uninterrupted sleep. I've supported parents who were so anxious, that they couldn't sleep out of fear that if they weren't watching, the baby might stop breathing. These parents essentially paid me to watch the baby breathe for them.

There are many reasons why parents might want support at night. These may or may not be a match for your priorities or scheduling preferences. As with the rest of your doula practice, your personal and professional boundaries frame your decision-making process.

The postpartum doula can help parents to learn the skill of flexibility by modeling it. If it is possible for the doula to offer a somewhat flexible schedule by adding shifts, cutting back, or changing times when appropriate, parents can learn that they will be the most successful by listening to their baby and working together, rather than trying to "schedule" their lives together. To be clear, flexibility does not mean that the doula should make themselves constantly available. Our own needs remain a priority. Anticipating needs for flexibility and how to best meet them for ourselves as well as our clients will make last-minute scheduling crisis an infrequent occurrence.

For parents hiring a doula prenatally, any scheduling agreed to is premature because the birth experience and outcome, as well as the personality of the baby, are not possible to anticipate. While it, of course, makes sense to set up a basic schedule, both doula and parents would do well to be prepared to make changes as the situation requires. This is one reason why working together with another doula, agency, or cooperative can be a working solution for both doula and parents.

What Might a Work Day be Like?

Here are some suggestions, assuming that you're there for a basic day shift. This is not intended to imply chronological order—just things you might do.

- ✓ Wash your hands upon arrival. Also, before preparing food, holding, or assisting with or feeding the baby.

- ✓ Make sure that the mother always has something to drink.

- ✓ Offer to make lunch or a snack. Always leave the kitchen tidy. Encourage parents to eat healthy meals by creating them.

- ✓ Help them to resource and strategize: meals for upcoming days, how to build a support community, strategies for creating sleep.

✓ Be prepared to make suggestions for ways you can help, if no tasks are requested.

✓ Make suggestions to ease adjustment.

✓ Encourage and compliment parents in doing things their own way. The doula is there to help them develop their own style.

✓ Listen to both parents (if there are two) as they describe how they're feeling. Serve as a safe place where they can try on different parenting ideas without being judged or instructed. Offer suggestions when asked, but remain open; remember, this is their baby.

✓ Model the art of supporting a mother during the postpartum period. Be prepared to offer ideas for what to expect and specific suggestions of how to help.

✓ Thirty minutes before leaving, begin to transition by preparing for your absence. Are parents and baby located where they will be comfortable for a while? Do they need anything? Do they have something to drink? Do they have any last-minute questions?

How Long Does the Postpartum Doula Spend With a Family?

Doula support can last anywhere from one or two visits to months. Any number of factors come into play in determining the duration of doula support. Considerations include:

What was the birth experience like?

Recovery from an uncomplicated vaginal birth may require less than recovery from a significant tear, episiotomy, or cesarean birth.

How is feeding going?

A baby experiencing challenges in latching, a client experiencing milk- supply challenges, or a baby having stomach troubles can derail the early weeks as a family.

What kind of support is available from family and friends?

Who is available to nurture the parents, as well as to educate and support? Are any support people knowledgeable about nursing, infant characteristics and care, and physical changes experienced by the mother?

The financial capacity to pay.

This is the deciding factor for many families. Not only are parents considering how much they can afford, but they are also doing so at a time when expenses are going up, with the addition of a baby (or two or three).

The number of new babies.

Multiples frequently require more "extra hands" than a singleton baby. Multiples may require more in terms of baby-holding, feeding, and organization, as well as additional challenges in finding time to rest.

Are there older siblings?

If there are school-aged children, it might be helpful for the doula to provide support during the afternoon hours when they arrive home needing nurture, movement, and help with homework. Dinner and baths can be an exhausting time with a new baby added to the process. Regardless of their age, doula support may help to ensure that older children don't feel neglected and help parents to avoid feeling overburdened.

Are there differences?

Babies or parents with physical or emotional needs outside of the typical, nursing problems, or premature infants can all contribute to longer-term relationships.

What is the client like? Are they feeling supported?

Clients who are less confident may need more time before they feel ready to phase out doula care. Personality comes into play here—different people have different needs. Challenges can include perinatal mental health, nursing, and relationship dynamics. Find ways to help clients gather support outside of the doula/client relationship by recommending specific nursing groups, parenting groups and classes, faith-based groups, and activities as an approach for boosting support.

Does the parent feel supported?

Regardless of what was anticipated and put into place, is it enough?

If there is a partner, do they feel supported?

Any parent, regardless of role or gender, may feel challenged in meeting everyone's needs while adjusting to parenthood.

Who is this baby?

Babies come with their personalities fully in place. Just like adults, some are more laid back and seem easier to please, while others are more challenged by adjusting to life on the outside or recovering from birth. Health concerns, prematurity, and sensitivity are all factors unique to the baby and cannot be predicted.

How Are Postpartum Doulas Paid?

New doulas are wise to research the financial aspect of the profession. The following information is based on the assumption that you will be self-employed as a doula.

Some commonly asked questions include:

How are doulas paid?

Most doulas charge for their services on an hourly basis. Some offer packages, in which the higher the number of support hours, the lower the hourly fee.

How much should I charge per hour?

This is completely up to you. Wages in any field are usually influenced by location and what you have to offer. Cost of living is a factor within any profession. Generally, wages are higher in communities with a higher cost of living. Experience can also be a determining factor. Some doula cooperatives offer "tiers," with experience and additional certifications as factors distinguishing different levels.

How do contracts work?

Most doulas work with contracts. You may choose as a doula to require your clients to commit upon hiring you to a particular schedule, including days of the week and exact hours. You may also have set standards for how long those shifts can or cannot be. You decide. As a doula, I have found that for me, flexibility matches my style best. I ask my clients to share what kind of support they anticipate needing, understanding that they won't really know for sure until the baby is born.

Flexibility has benefits, because it allows the new family to receive the support that they need based on the real situation: not what they anticipated. However, flexibility means greater stress on the doula, who may find that they have more (or less) work than anticipated with a particular family. Working with a community of doulas allows for accommodation. If you are working on your own, your contract should reflect this, to include your approach to overlapping families. Any approach is fine as long as it works for you and your clients. As you gain experience, expect your contract to evolve. Again, you will have to look into yourself and ask, "What are my priorities? What will work for me? What do my clients need?" and act accordingly.

Do I charge the same amount regardless of the number of hours or the time of day?

Once again, this is up to you. Some doulas set it up as the more hours purchased, the less the clients pay per hour. Essentially, it's buying in bulk. Doulas also sometimes charge more for overnights or for families with multiples. Again, there are benefits and drawbacks. What sounds right to you?

How much can I expect to earn?

Of course, everyone needs to know the bottom line. The answer to this is a pretty straightforward formula. Decide how much you will charge hourly. Determine what your expenses will be (education, certification costs, marketing, transportation, phone bills, professional liability insurance, printing costs, and taxes, to name a few). Determine how many hours you can or need to work in a week. Multiply desired hours worked by the amount you will charge. This will give you a general idea of your gross (pre-tax) income. Next, factor out your expenses. This will provide you with a picture of your potential financial situation. Then get out there and find the work!

Do I Have to be a Parent to be Effective?

No! At the core, a doula needs a willing heart and hands. Next, follow education, experience with babies, information, and referrals to offer clients as situations arise. Doulas do not need to have birthed or raised children of their own to possess these qualifications.

A person who has had children of their own may have the benefit of familiarity with newborns and skills, such as diaper changing and burping, but this only goes so far. Immersed in an infant-rich environment, it quickly becomes clear that once you've successfully changed ten or so diapers, you have developed competency, if not yet expertise. The same can be said for burping or swaddling: these skills are easily learned. They will also need to be adapted to the preferences and needs of each individual baby and family that you support. The essence of doula care is much less concrete. It's not just what we know but how we convey that knowledge that differentiates our support, subtle tips and acceptance, and extensive resources.

The person who feels better prepared to be a doula because of personal experience as a parent may not offer the flexible, non-judgmental support parents are hoping for. This is because that person may not recognize how limited their own experience really is. For example, a parent of three healthy singleton babies may have never:

- ✓ Nursed

- ✓ Nursed multiples

- ✓ Formula-fed

- ✓ Cared for a baby with a disability

- ✓ Single parented

- ✓ Experienced challenging relationships with a partner or others in the home

- ✓ Parented a baby with severe reflux problems

- ✓ Experienced long-term breastfeeding challenges

- ✓ Parented a baby born prematurely, requiring a lengthy hospital stay

- ✓ Experienced the loss of a baby

- ✓ Experienced a perinatal mood disorder

- ✓ Recovered from a cesarean

No doula has experienced all that their clients will. We should all arrive prepared to adapt to each and every situation. These are skills that are not contingent upon parenting experience.

Additional FAQ

How should I dress to work as a doula?

You are an individual, with your own style and tastes. These should be reflected in your dress as a doula. Aim for the intersection of comfort and professionalism. Ideally, you will wear clothing that is neat and clean while projecting your own style and concept of the profession. As with any other job, most people dress up more for an interview than they do for every other day of work.

If you dress over-casually, your role may be perceived as one of physical labor than professional support. For example, a person in sweats might be perceived as expecting to do the house cleaning. Strive to find a balance between durability, washability (remember, these clothes may get spit-up upon), and a professional appearance. All in all, this is about you, how you perceive your role, and how you choose to present yourself. As with all other choices, you have the ability to change your approach in this area at any time. Be you. And then be the next you, if a new you arises.

Things to avoid:

✓ Scratchy clothes.

✓ Clothes that need to be dry-cleaned.

✓ Jewelry that could poke at a baby when you are holding them close.

✓ Perfume and other scents

✓ Scrubs. Whether they're green or colorful with bunnies and bears, these were developed for medical personnel, and they come with expectations and sometimes authority messages. Doulas are completely non-medical.

On Driving and Cooking

Should I drive the children to school, or parents to doctor's appointments?

There are no rules or policies on this in a legal sense. That said, there are factors that may leave the doula wary of taking on these roles due to potential insurance and liability considerations. If you own a car, check with your insurance company to determine if you would be covered while driving as a doula. Alternatively, the doula can ride along in the car to help parents with the baby and other children.

What kind of foods should I cook?

This will depend on the needs and preferences of the families that you support. Three priorities to keep in mind are nutrition, safety, and culture. Make a point of learning about these, both in general and as they relate to your individual clients. Learn about nutrition, especially the needs of a mother during the postpartum period. Ask your clients if they follow any specific dietary rules or if anyone in the home has any food allergies.

Do I have to cook?

If you are not comfortable preparing meals, be sure your potential clients understand that it is not something that you offer. Or perhaps you are comfortable with assembling food—making a salad or sandwich rather than cooking. As long as clients understand this upfront, they are able to select their doula according to their own preferences.

I enjoy cooking, and I am vegetarian/am vegan/keep kosher/other

If you are not comfortable preparing meat or any other food, just let your clients know. See above.

Do I have to do everything asked? Do I have to stay, no matter what?

No! Your personal and professional boundaries will guide your practice—ideally, up-front and in advance, so your role is clear to all. Some things will be more straightforward to share in advance:

- ✓ Your role in general terms
- ✓ Hours you work
- ✓ How/when you expect to be paid
- ✓ How/when to communicate with you

These can all be described in your written materials, your contract, and on your website.

Other things can be more challenging to articulate:

- ✓ Your role as it relates to parenting practices
- ✓ How you expect to be treated
- ✓ How you expect others to be treated

You may choose to design policies on these and review them with clients in written form. If you find this challenging, it's not surprising. You are walking a line between ensuring respectful treatment (of yourself, of the newborn, of older children) and sounding like a rigid person who perhaps is expecting worst of people. It is impossible to anticipate every type of interaction that could be triggering or challenging, and trying to express them all in written form could lose you potential clients, while still not covering every possible eventuality. Even if you are unable to find a way to positively phrase your expectations in written form, it is worth expressing them through conversation during your intake visit, as well as in a casual, respectful manner as appropriate throughout your time with a family.

While it is our role to support our clients non-judgmentally and honor their choices, we do not need to compromise our standards of how we expect ourselves or others to be treated, to include taking part in parenting practices we consider to be developmentally inappropriate or antithetical to the way we see the roles of parents and ourselves. Not every support person will be a match for every family. When these situations arise (which should happen infrequently if you are careful with your intakes and communication of your role), express your concerns in a nonjudgmental manner and suggest that a different doula would be a better support match.

Should You Certify? Why? With Which Organization(s)?

As the profession of doula support spreads both geographically and in terms of acceptance, legal requirements have the potential to change rapidly. In places where doulas are unlicensed, meaning there is no governmental body setting standards for doula training and conduct, we are off the governmental radar (except for taxes, of course). As a practicing or aspiring doula, this is an aspect of research you'll want to keep on top of. Until licensure is required, doulas are vulnerable in the same ways that people in any other profession are. For example, there are laws regarding business practices; anyone can get into trouble for falsely representing their services, their qualifications, or by stealing. Anyone can also find themselves in trouble for practicing medicine without a license. For this reason, we need to conduct our practice within our role. Dabbling in clinical skills, such as diagnosing and treating conditions, can be a slippery slope, especially for doulas, who are offering their services in a professional capacity. The situation above is our reality and unless doulas are regulated (which creates its own set of challenges and setbacks), certification is the option available to us in terms of setting standards of practice and ethics that will protect both doulas and the families that they serve.

Certification offers a standard of practice and professional moral compass, and for many, it serves as an excellent launching point. It can offer the new doula clarification of the role and bring them to a standard that is sometimes higher than what an individual might have the foresight to consider. For these reasons, it is the starting point for many doulas. So, how do you choose what organization to certify through?

The answer: research, just as you will encourage your clients to do. Identify your priorities and goals. Thoroughly research the organizations you're considering. Are they for-profit or non-profit? What is their history? Who is their leadership? What is their vision? Does their definition and depiction of doula support gel with your vision of yourself as a doula and what families need? What do they offer you in terms of ongoing education, resources, and reputation? What standards do they hold doulas to in terms of accountability, and is there a practice in place for grievances from clients, doulas, or other professionals? In what ways do they promote doulas?

Cost is obviously a consideration, as is convenience. By convenience, I am referencing time and finances invested in the process. Sometimes these are the primary considerations—people want to be certified, and they want to be certified quickly so they can get to the work of supporting families. This is a valid priority but shouldn't be the only one.

The organization you choose to certify through will likely set your core priorities and practices. It also sends a message to prospective clients, doulas, and other professionals. Be certain that you are choosing an organization that matches who you want to be as a doula.

Certification—Additional Considerations

Are there downsides to certification? Not in and of themselves, but there are factors to consider that can offer decision-making data points.

The first thing to keep in mind is to remember that in many places, there is no regulation of doula certifying organizations. This means that you (or your brother or your neighbor) could open a corporation and begin certifying doulas tomorrow, and there would be nothing illegal about it. It may be unethical, but it is legal, so take the time to investigate the program you are considering. Consider the questions listed previously and your own priorities. Is it important that it be a non-profit? Working together with other organizations toward change? Only you can answer these questions. Keep in mind that you are a consumer and make yourself an educated one.

Compatibility is another main point to consider. Again, it requires research: is the organization aligned with your priorities? Are the standards of practice compatible with the way you plan to conduct yourself?

For example, some organizations offer standards limiting the use of herbs or homeopathy by doulas due to the role being non-clinical. If this is incompatible with your plans due to your own beliefs or areas of additional training, why certify and then practice in contradiction of documents that you have signed? Find another organization that it a closer match. Alternatively, take the training but do not certify. When potential clients ask if you are certified, you can explain that you are trained through X organization, but not certified by choice, for the following reasons. People almost always react well to a situation in which you are taking your reasoning to an even higher level. Anyone who chooses otherwise likely would not have been a match either way.

Other Voices for
Professional Doulas

Birdsong Brooklyn—A Doula Partnership Story

As an educator, I have been blessed to train hundreds of doulas each year for almost 20 years. It's a blessing because each attendee has also been a teacher, and I have been able to soak up their wisdom and pass it along to the next generations of doulas who pass through my workshops.

It is important to me that *Nurturing the Family* include voices other than mine. In planning, I felt strongly that I wanted to include the voices of doulas who were still immersed in the building of their businesses, to bring fresh eyes and perspective.

Erica and Laura attended my doula workshop together, and from the first hour, I was struck by their insight, ability to engage, and the power of the friendship that was now about to blossom into a working partnership as well. I could tell that these friends were going places in the doula world, and today, I can say that I was right. I asked them to answer some basic questions on doula work. Enjoy.

The Voices of Birdsong Brooklyn

by Laura Interlandi and Erica Livingston

When training in New York, Jackie often asked us to speak to the newly trained postpartum doulas. It's one of our favorite things to do and we always get so excited to meet them and speak with them. We end with a Q and A, and participants ask us questions that make us think deeply about why we do this and how we can all always be growing and getting better. So when Jackie asked us to co-write a chapter we were over the moon about the idea. Being able to be guest speakers for everyone who reads this book is a dream.

FAQ from New Doulas

Why did you become postpartum doulas?

Picture the scene—prenatal yoga, Brooklyn. Laura had spent the morning writing positive affirmations about finding a friend and as class opened, right beside her sat Erica. We struck up a conversation: we were reading the same book, planning similar births and both wondered how to balance art and motherhood. Without knowing it, Erica played out the role of postpartum doula: sitting with Laura postbirth, holding her baby girl while she showered, making her tea and food and doing her dishes. Three months later, when it was Erica's turn, both of us were even better equipped and educated. We marveled at what an incredible difference even the smallest amount of support made.

As the weeks and months continued we found ourselves in tender disbelief—where would we have been without each other? How do new parents not have this? How is this not the norm? Postpartum support is as vital as birth support. With the advent of birth doulas and more educated and empowered birth choices surely there was room for better postpartum experiences also? Of course, we obsess over birth. It is amazing. Birth is exciting, sexy, transformative and follows a narrative that pleases us. Postpartum however, is messy, decidedly UNsexy and seriously lacking in resources, dialogue and visibility. There was clearly a gap in the dialogue, we realized, and our calling was to fill it. And so began Birdsong Brooklyn.

Primary message: If you are a doula, you are a business and your product is yourself. Treat it as a business. Take that part as seriously as you do the role and learning about birthing families because if you don't, it will remain a hobby and never be a career. This book isn't focused on marketing and promoting yourself as a professional; rather the premise is to begin to equip you to work as a doula so that you have a skill to market. The lack of focus on this subject matter should not translate into a lack of emphasis on this aspect of your work. In fact, the reason why it's not covered is that it's so enormous. Read the chapter on doula business skills as a very basic launching point. Then it'll be time to really get started. On an ongoing basis, you should do the following (marketing specific):

- ✓ Take classes
- ✓ Listen to podcasts
- ✓ Join supportive groups online
- ✓ Take online classes
- ✓ Read books
- ✓ Build relationships with doulas and other professionals that serve the same clients as you do
- ✓ Learn about taxes
- ✓ Give back to your community
- ✓ Learn about local business requirements
- ✓ Learn about record keeping

How do you juggle doula work and life?

In any kind of freelance life there are periods of overload and times that are leaner. For us it is imperative to work together, sharing clients where possible, backing each other or serving as one another's processor. In the beginning we shared childcare of our little ones, and while challenging, it was the jumping off point we needed and addressed the block we were having as we worked towards a level of experience and rate of pay that afforded quality care. There is tremendous work to be done growing and maintaining a business beyond the time spent with a client. Sharing the load makes it all seem possible.

It is also so important to model self care to your clients. Having a baseline of reserve energy from which to practice is ideal- then if a great opportunity floods in you have a well to draw from. If you are constantly working on empty, your work will not be of quality. YOU are your product.

This is a career path that requires communication skills that can only truly be accessed in the present moment. Active listening and conscious communication is what is required at all times, but it's hard to do sometimes..

What's your business model?

The short answer: It is fluid and sprawling.

Long Answer: We have tried different approaches and suspect we will continue to move with the needs of our own families, clients, selves and opportunities that come. When we began, we shared clients 50/50 and also traded childcare to make working possible. Our kids were 8 and 5 months when we did our doula training and 10 and 7 months when we landed our first paying client. We worked for that client Tues/Thurs 10-2 for 12 weeks. One of us would stay with the babes and the other would go to work, and the next day we would switch. This worked for a while. But as our kiddos were growing up, we both felt more comfortable with outside childcare and we raised our rates to accommodate that. It helped our business and around that time we both had long contract clients requesting almost full time care and so we split for a while to accommodate those needs.

Now we serve as one another's back up where possible. We even had a 1 day/week nanny share at one point, that assured a regular time slot to offer a client or for us to meet and discuss what is going on business wise. Sometimes one of us wants to take on more work while the other wishes to pare down- we came to realize that the more flexible we were willing to be with each other and our business model, the more balance we could strike and the more likely we could continue to truly love this work without burning out. Positive, clear communication is key in managing expectations with your partner. Laura recently re-structured her life to live part time in Canada which has been yet another structural overhaul. This shift has required a deeper commitment to our goals, communication and a creative nimbleness to meet our deadlines and stay aligned.

There is of course an "on call" aspect to our job, even more so that now we also take occasional birth and full spectrum clients. If a postpartum family is struggling early on and we can accommodate a spur of the moment shift we will try our best to do so. But we work with a contract in place and one of our conditions is that scheduling must be locked down 24hrs before a desired visit, and we also require payment before we arrive. We have learned this the hard way. For the clients that hire us prenatally, we require them to book a package of hours (20 minimum) and pay at least a 50% deposit up front. For these clients we also schedule a 4hr prenatal that comes out of their package. Although it initially sounds like a lot, 4 hours flies by. We cover everything: postpartum healing,infant feeding, babywearing, meal prep and a getting to know you that covers the clients desires and also the practical ways their home and space functions. We take notes, write down their questions and afterwards create a google doc that we continue to work with throughout our time. Since we started requiring the prenatal we have had overall better outcomes, happier clients and an easier time navigating the home and family dynamics. The client then has 4 four hour shifts which usually we rotate visits.

Before the second postpartum visit we require they pay the remainder of the fee. By the last shift we will have discussed whether more hours are desired, and a new transaction takes place to begin a new package of hours. We have found that the more upfront we are about money, contracts and logistics the easier it flows. There is nothing worse than having to disturb a postpartum client having an emotional day to ask for a check at the end of your shift—well except maybe not being able to pay your rent!

There are, of course, times when clients find us after baby is born and have a specific area of need or time they want from us. Perhaps someone just needs 2-3 visits while their partner is out of town. We discuss on the phone and explain our packages, decide on a number of hours, send them a contract and ask for a deposit or full payment on the time they think they want. Clients must understand that scheduling preferences go to those who request it in advance and are paid up.

In addition to one-to-one doula work we create original curriculum for parenting and birthworker themed workshops that we teach around the city and online. We blog, run social media, speak at events and meetups, host community gatherings and ceremonies, operate a formal 13 week global online mentorship program called SEEN, and offer consulting/corporate training. There are infinite ways to use your knowledge of postpartum, and the world needs all of them. The more successful you are, the more healing happens. We want things to change faster for more parents than we can serve on a one-to-one level; we encourage new doulas to first ground themselves in the work but to also stay open and think outside the box. That is the beauty and creativity of being an entrepreneur.

What's your best advice for new doulas?

Be open to being changed by this work while protecting your heart. Postpartum is a raw and vulnerable time. The birthing person is a portal, wide open and slowly healing. Intense things can happen, take time for yourself (even 5 minutes) right before and after a shift to nourish yourself and let go of anything you are carrying from your own life or from theirs. Know your power but also its limits. You are not there to save anyone, you are not the hero (your client is!) even though sometimes you feel like it (and it's great when you do!). How you feel after a shift isn't always indicative of how good of a job you did. They are paying you to not have to say thank you or manage your emotions. They can have a hard day and be direct with you.

You may experience the best shift you ever did but you may feel completely worn out. You may only get that thank you on babe's first birthday with a card in the mail, or never at all. Be self-affirming. Holding space is a learned skill and also an inherent gift. Know your strengths and also work to continue to expand your limitations. You cannot be all things to all people, but you can be the most compassionate, educated and professional YOU.

Be yourself at interviews. Not everyone will hire you but when they do they will hire you because they genuinely like you, your vibe and what you are offering, which will be so much easier and more fun as you work with them. It will also garner you more and better aligned referrals. Seek mentorship and community. Get a partner or at least a back-up. Have fun. And if you aren't naturally a funny person, take an improv class, learn some jokes or call us! People need to laugh postpartum! There are so many bodily fluids you've just got to laugh.

What's your favorite thing about this work?

Watching a new parent acknowledge themself as powerful and exactly everything their baby needs. Seeing them grow into their role and reclaim pieces of themself as they assume a new identity: bearing witness to nothing short of full transformation. We love watching the light return to their eyes, cheeks flush with color after a good meal. Our reward is that moment when they text us a picture, wearing their baby and smiling proudly.

Holding the space for a family to make the choices they want to make and feel educated and confident (and maybe even rested, ha!) gives us a feeling like no other. Seeing families thrive is one of our favorite things in this world.

NURTURING THE FAMILY

The Business Side of Doula Work
by Patty Brennan

Have you ever hired a contractor to work on your home? You know, the guy who has great carpentry and plumbing skills? He can do anything you need. Except show up on time, meet a deadline, or communicate effectively about his prices, or what's even involved in the job. I've fired five accountants, three website designers, one graphic artist, and multiple housing-related contractors. The reason for this is that most folks who are self-employed do not have the full skill set they need to run their businesses. They think that because they have a specialized skill set, that in itself makes them an asset. They are wrong.

Attending doula training and completing the professional certification process are just the beginning steps of building a viable doula business. Serving families well is the heart and soul of your work—your reason for being a doula. It is what you love. But the rest of it, creating the infrastructure for building your business, establishing and communicating your value, staying out of trouble with taxes, managing liability, and getting the word out are also essential pieces. All entrepreneurs—and if you are in business for yourself, you are an entrepreneur—need to work on their business, not just in their business. This takes time and commitment. It might not be your favorite part of your job, but overlook this skill set at your peril because you will just be another struggling person for whom self-employment translates to underemployment or, worse yet, unemployment. Bottom line, you can't help moms and babies if you need a paycheck and you can't pay yourself.

When I first came to birth work as a childbirth educator, doula, and aspiring homebirth midwife, I was a self-employed, working mother of two. I decided that self-employment suited me, and I have never changed my mind on that score. Most of the skills I acquired from running my business easily transferred to birth work, and I found that I had a leg up on many of the new friends I came to know in birth circles, some of whom were struggling to be paid for their work. In the intervening years, my work has evolved significantly. I have founded a thriving childbirth education and doula training center, as well as two nonprofit doula programs, and have trained over 2,000 doulas. As a close observer of our profession, I believe I have a unique insight into common mistakes made and the challenges faced by passionate new doulas who are also new to the business side of things.

So, do you have what it takes to make it? That fire in your belly is a great start! You can build on that, and it is just possible you may discover that the dreaded business side is actually not so bad. Building a successful business is a multifaceted creative process that will bring a multitude of skills into play. Some of them will be your strong suit. Others, not so much. Just remember, you can always acquire new skills, educate yourself in areas that are new to you, and, when necessary, outsource some tasks to specialists. None of this happens overnight.

Communication Skills

Both verbal and written communication skills are important. Undoubtedly, doula-listening skills were covered in your core doula training. These are important, as they will help you stay within your scope of practice and enable families to problem-solve their own issues with nonjudgmental support. If you ever have the opportunity to take training in Motivational Interviewing, I highly recommend it. Motivational Interviewing is similar to reflective listening but more subtle and nuanced. It will make you a better doula.

Business communication is different. Whether written or verbal, it is not subtle or nuanced, but rather focused and clear. Writing skills are needed to create your contract for services and other client paperwork, as well as all of your promotional materials, including rack cards, ads, social media posts, press releases, and content for your website. Spelling and grammatical errors are unacceptable and will undermine your professional image. Can you be a great doula and a poor speller? Absolutely! Can you convince potential customers to trust you if your rack card, website, or email communications have glaring errors? Perhaps a few will overlook this failing, but many will be turned off. The key here is to be self-aware. Get help if you need it, even if you don't think you need it (a special conceit that few can live up to), use spellcheck programs, and have a competent reviewer go over your stuff before going public with it. Sometimes we can't "see" what we have written because we have lost all perspective after multiple rewritings. A fresh set of eyes will see what we can't and, hopefully, invite us to question our assumptions as well.

Setting and Maintaining Professional Boundaries

Those of us in the helping professions are uniquely challenged in this regard, given the intimate and heart-centered nature of our work. Still, when someone is paying you for a professional service, you are not their friend, no matter how much you may enjoy working together. You are being paid to be a really good listener, to be supportive, and to meet their needs.

The scope of practice for doulas should help with setting boundaries— there are simply some things that doulas do not do. Your client contract is a tool for setting boundaries and communicating them to your clients, and trial and error will lead you to setting new boundaries when you find yourself uncomfortably on the wrong side of where the line needs to be drawn. That's normal. How else are you going to know how many clients you can comfortably take on in a given timeframe? When you are at the beginning, a bit of guesswork is involved and then you simply keep refining it over time.

Once boundaries are established, we must be prepared to maintain our boundaries when (not if) they are challenged. This is a skill, and it gets easier with practice. If you find that your clients are repeatedly not respecting your boundaries, for example, not paying you on time or expecting services outside of your contract, try to be curious about why this keeps happening. Did you give mixed signals, somehow undermining your own boundaries? Did you tell the woman on the phone that your initial consultation would take one hour, but then you spent two with her and her partner? Make sure, going forward, that there is congruency between your expectations and your actions, and I guarantee that you will find that maintaining boundaries gets easier.

Building Relationships

Also known as professional networking, relationship building is essential to your success as a doula. One key relationship that becomes a steady source of referrals can make the difference between success and failure. Cultivate several solid referral sources, and you will have all the work you can handle. When networking, remember that all successful relationships are two-way streets, so think about ways to reciprocate and bring value to your referral partners as well.

Ethical Behavior

No one can truly succeed in this field if they are not upholding ethical business standards. Transparency is key. Put simply, this means no surprises. You need to deliver on what you have promised to the client. Ethical guidelines for doulas have been thoughtfully and thoroughly articulated by most certifying agencies. Compliance with these guidelines is required of certified doulas and strongly encouraged for all practicing doulas.

Money-Management Skills

Basic bookkeeping is required of anyone who is self-employed. At a minimum, a system for tracking income and expenses needs to be in place. This can be as simple as purchasing and using a two-column ledger book from the local office supply store or as complicated as setting up a chart of accounts in QuickBooks that will enable you to track everything online. You will also want to track mileage for business use of your vehicle.

There is more to the money-management side of running a business than setting up a bookkeeping system. In order to make money, you must be prepared to strategically invest in your business—spend money in order to make it, as the saying goes. Failure to develop a website, for example, will substantially limit your success. So, the ability to forecast income and expenses, set priorities, and create a budget for your business is also necessary.

Marketing Skills

This is a whole realm unto itself, with multiple components. No one has it down because the world is constantly changing, and our message, as well as how we deliver it, is also essentially fluid. You need to become a student of marketing. Read books, follow some of the marketing gurus (e.g., Seth Godin), take a class, join a marketing or mastermind group. Engage.

I was prejudiced against marketing for many years, feeling it was somewhat tainted or unworthy. Isn't it enough to be a really great doula and create good word of mouth about my services? Must I really sell myself? As I learned more about what marketing truly is, I began to reframe my view and to understand that marketing is, at its core, education. Education about the value of the doula's role. Marketing answers the question in the consumer's mind, "Why should I care?" Further, it makes the case why you are the best choice among all of their choices in the marketplace. What value do you bring to families? What is unique about you? This is the case you need to make. Generally, people are not as price resistant as we might imagine; they just don't want to think they are spending their money stupidly.

Time-Management Skills

This is perhaps one of the most useful skills of all. Being your own boss and setting your own schedule certainly offer a welcome degree of flexibility and freedom in life. But if flexibility comes to mean a complete lack of discipline in devoting time to work on your business, then you will find that you don't have a viable business. Try to block some time each week to work on your business and follow a plan or organized approach (as outlined in goal setting below).

Goal-Setting Abilities

They say that "the difference between a dream and a goal is a deadline." Yup. Set a goal and a deadline. Next, work backward from the deadline to sketch out the action steps necessary to achieve your goal. Each of the action steps will also require a deadline. Next, work the plan. If you find that you are struggling with staying on track, get an accountability partner, and set regular check-in times with each other. If you are feeling stuck and not making the progress you anticipated, then your accountability partner can help you determine what supports you may need to keep moving forward. Then, make a new plan and work it.

Five Traps for Aspiring Doula Entrepreneurs

1. Limiting Beliefs about Money

There seems to be a widespread belief that making money and doing work one loves are irreconcilable goals. I have heard many variations on the theme, "I don't want money to be my focus." This statement is often followed by a "but..." The notion that financial success is incompatible with being a doula is a false dichotomy. How about this instead? "I love my job as a doula, AND I love being well paid for it." No buts, apologies, or justifications required. In fact, if one aims to live a fulfilling life, absolutely loving what you spend the bulk of your time doing is the key. If you continually find yourself slipping into this false dichotomy, you will need to reprogram your beliefs about money.

Why do doulas share a tendency to undervalue our important contributions to a family's wellbeing? As doulas, we are professionalizing a role that has been performed willingly by women throughout time and across all cultures, typically without reimbursement. There have always been women like us—those who feel a special calling, and have a special talent for, helping mothers when their babies are born and through the early weeks postpartum. Support at this time is needed and, historically, has been provided outside of the flow of commerce. It is understandable that many modern doulas feel guilty charging money for services that are so obviously needed, so basic to a family's well-being.

We must not fall into this trap. Previously undervalued "women's work" has emerged as an integral part of our modern economy. When a new mother is successful with breastfeeding, healthcare dollars are saved, and working mothers miss fewer days of work due to caring for sick children. Likewise, the provision of essential postpartum support services can reduce the number of return visits to the ER for both the mom and baby. Problems may be prevented altogether, obviating the need for medical intervention, or caught early and appropriate non-urgent referrals made. And, while quantitative research that firmly establishes the financial benefits to society of postpartum doula work is needed, the truth resonates in each of us.

Embrace and celebrate the value that you bring to families. Working for little-to-no money while calling oneself a professional doula undervalues our profession as a whole. A little reprogramming may be called for here. As an exercise in self-worth, list every benefit of a postpartum doula you can think of. Next, list every asset you bring to the table. This can include personal experience, character, and strengths, as well as professional training, skills, and experience. Post this where you can see it several times a day until you have fully integrated it into your self-talk, language, and beliefs. If you still find yourself feeling guilty about your fees on occasion, be curious about the beliefs that underlie your guilt. Name them. Where do they come from? How can you rewrite your own script? How can you bring great value to each family whom you serve?

2. Sense of Entitlement

Completing doula training and certification is simply the first step on the doula career path. It is a jumping-off point for creating a career. Some folks, however, seem to have unrealistic expectations that, after training, they will immediately start generating income as a doula. I have had students express disappointment, frustration, and discouragement when their expectations are not met. However, when questioned closely, I learn that they have done very little to promote their services, get the word out about their business, or make professional connections in the community. Essentially, they seem to have expected prospective customers to raise their hands or somehow know to knock on their door. It is akin to a person who complains about being lonely and not having friends but then sits home weekend after weekend watching TV. That's not how it works. So, stop feeling sorry for yourself. Stop expecting everything to magically land in your lap and accept responsibility for charting your own course. You are the captain of your own ship. Henry Ford had a great quote (it was about men, so I have to change it as follows): "One [woman] thinks [she] can, and one [woman] thinks [she] can't. They're both right."

3. Misunderstanding Marketing

There are three integrated aspects to marketing: (1) the market, (2) your message, and (3) the media. Knowing your market requires you to have in mind a clear picture of your ideal customer. Customer demographics are one aspect of this picture, but you need to dig a little deeper. What do your customers care about? What problems do they have that you can help solve? Your message needs to be carefully crafted to your ideal customer, speaking to their concerns, and resonating emotionally with them. What do they need? What motivates them?

Let's consider your rack card as an example. For too many of us, our print media boils down to a list of services provided (albeit in a pretty package). Even just changing the heading "Available Services" to "Ways I Can Help Your Family" would be heading in the right direction. Your message is not about you; it is about them. This is an important filter to have in place because our tendency is to frame our services in terms of what we are offering. Why should anyone care that you provide postpartum doula services or do placental encapsulation?

Finally, we need to choose the best media to deliver our message to our target market. There is a wide range of methods for getting your message out.

Try to diversify your approach rather than becoming overly reliant upon just one funnel, like your website, for example. Think in terms of print media (rack cards, flyers, business cards, published articles, directory, and calendar listings); venues (exhibitor tables at baby fairs, health fairs, conferences, and trade shows); events and public speaking; networking with other professionals to generate referrals; and online media (blog, social media, e-newsletters). As you try different approaches, attempt to build in a way of tracking their effectiveness so that you can measure the return on your investment of both time and money.

4. The House of Cards

One approach to creating a successful business is to focus on careful cultivation of a business model and clientele, and grow organically from the ground up. This is a relatively low-risk way to proceed. Contrast this approach with the grandiose but underfunded (high-risk) business visionary. This person has no problem seeing herself as an entrepreneur. She is creative, ambitious, and hard-working. She wants it all, and she wants it now. Perhaps she has some family money to invest, or maybe she goes into debt. Her vision is to have a center where moms and babies come together for classes, services, support groups, and perhaps retail. She signs a lease for commercial property and invests money, time, and energy designing and furnishing the space. She brainstorms an impressive list of programs, classes, and mother-baby groups and crafts a mission statement. Now she is the proud owner of the best-kept secret in town. It's a house of cards, and unless our visionary also quickly becomes a savvy marketer, her top-down model is in danger of collapsing.

Here's an example of someone doing it right. A stay-at-home mom who is a cloth diaper enthusiast discovers an unmet need in her community. She opens a cloth diaper business from her home. Eventually, this business outgrows her home, and she rents inexpensive office space off the beaten track in order to increase her inventory and regain her family's privacy. Gradually, she adds other specialized baby products to her inventory and moves to a storefront in a busy shopping mall. Over the course of these years, she is acquiring a loyal customer base and new skills. Each expansion is supported by market demand, and her overall risk is minimal.

A little patience and thoughtful persistence are called for. Common wisdom tells us it takes a minimum of three years for a new business venture to become viable.

5. Lack of a Plan

There are so many aspects to running a business, tasks to be completed, and skills to acquire, that it is easy to become overwhelmed. And that overwhelm can turn into immobilization. My friend, a freelance writer, calls it "dusting the blinds syndrome" when he procrastinates working by allowing himself to be distracted by just about anything. He's up for grabs, so to speak. Articulating your goals and creating a plan will help make a daunting project doable. It just needs to be broken down into bite-size pieces. Deadlines are your friend. To revert to my being-the-captain-of-our-own-ship metaphor, do captains sail forth without knowing where they are going, how they are getting there, and when they expect to arrive? Do they just drift aimlessly or do they chart a course? And which method (drifting or planning) do you think is more likely to get you to your destination?

Nine Questions for Start-Ups

Your answers to the nine start-up questions are foundational for your business. Once you have carefully considered your answers, you are ready to draw up your client contract or letter of agreement. You also have, by the way, just developed content for the services page on your website and are now ready to handle calls from clients seeking services. *Voila*!

1. What will you name your business?

This is a more complex process than you might imagine. There are a number of considerations. Is it a good name? Is the name, or a close approximation of it, available as a URL for your website? Is it available in your state if you decide to incorporate (or is someone else already using it)? Have you integrated keywords in your name that will help folks searching for a postpartum doula to find you online? What do others think about your business name? Once you've settled it, buy the URL, even if you don't plan on developing a website right away.

2. Under what type of business structure do you plan to operate?

If you want to keep everything as simple as possible, you can go with the default choice of sole proprietor. However, there may be compelling reasons for you to become a limited liability corporation (LLC), S corporation, or nonprofit corporation. Perhaps you are considering establishing a doula partnership, a doula collective, or a doula agency? Each of these will have pros and cons that require careful deliberation. See *The Doula Business Guide* for more information.

3. What services are you offering?

Are there services that clients may be seeking from a postpartum doula that you exclude (e.g., house cleaning, dog walking, babysitting)? Be specific here. You may or may not want to communicate in writing everything excluded, but at least be clear in your own mind where the boundaries are.

4. What is your fee for services?

Before settling on a fee, do a little homework, and investigate the local doula scene. What are others charging? What is the range, and where do you fit in? The bottom line is you need to feel comfortable with your fee, be able to state it without apology, and believe in your heart that you are worth every penny. Typically, inexperienced doulas will place themselves at the lower end of the price continuum. As your knowledge and skills grow, so too will your confidence and your fee.

5. A few additional money-related details need to be considered.

What is your timeframe for payment of the fee? Do you require a deposit for reserving time in your schedule for clients (and potentially turning away other customers)? Is the deposit nonrefundable? If not, what is your refund policy? How will you accept payment? Should checks be made out to you personally or to your business name? If you incorporate, you will need a separate business checking account. If you are operating as a sole proprietor and accept checks made out to the business name, you will need to procure a DBA (doing business as) from your local county clerk's office. The DBA can then be added to your personal checking account so that checks made out to the business can be deposited directly to your personal account or you can opt to open a business account.

6. How far are you willing to travel?

If your radius is a generous one-hour travel time, keep in mind that the two hours on the road are uncompensated time. If you are considering shift work, for example, serving one client in the morning and another in the afternoon, then the travel radius will be a determining factor in your ability to manage multiple clients simultaneously.

7. How busy do you want to be?

What is your ideal number of work hours per week? What are the limits here, and how flexible can you be? Admittedly, the answer to this question may be difficult to predict. Just give it your best guess for now and realize that trial and error, as well as shifting circumstances and needs in your personal life, will likely guide your boundary setting as you go along.

8. Where will you meet with clients for the initial consultation?

In the case of postpartum doulas, my strong recommendation is that it should be in their home. This will give you a much better feel for them as a family, as well as an opportunity to directly experience the environment in which you are agreeing to provide services.

9. What are your backup arrangements, if any?

While postpartum doulas do not have the same critical need for backup that birth doulas do, I still recommended that you have help available to step in, should you become unable to fulfill your commitment to a family.

As for the nitty-gritty basics and detailed instructions on how to set up a limited liability corporation, meet basic bookkeeping and tax standards, create a website or optimize your website for the search engines, these topics (and a whole lot more) are covered in detail in my book, *The Doula Business Guide*, and its companion workbook. Cultivate the entrepreneur within you and, step-by-step, you CAN create a successful professional doula business. Happy trails!

On the Experiences and Support Needs of Families

Composing a Family

"Today, the materials and skills from which a life is composed are no longer clear. It is no longer possible to follow the paths of previous generations" (Bateson, 2001). In *Composing a Life*, Bateson also remarks that, "This is a book about life as an improvisatory art, about the ways we combine familiar and unfamiliar components in response to new situations [...]»

I believe the same holds true with the addition of a baby. A new person has joined the family, and adjustments will unfold organically through a series of reactions. Recently, I was exploring the idea of *composing* a family. Where would the differences be? For me, the difference is intention. Not intricate planning, not creating an unrealistic and unattainable concept of what life will be, but living intentionally as a family. Doulas can facilitate composing a family considering the needs of each person and how they weave into existing and new relationships, being flexibile as a practice, and reconsidering and making changes as situations evolve.

Along with the joy and relief that arrive with a new baby, we can also find fatigue, stress, and jealousy. Remain sensitive to the needs of all family members and how their lives have changed. Siblings have been displaced. They may feel confused—or even abandoned. The doula can help by offering them much needed attention and by freeing up some of their parents' time.

Mothers are experiencing a transition. Even with a wanted baby, a supportive partner, no breastfeeding challenges, and feeling emotionally healthy, the new mother still faces difficulties. Mothers are tired; they are often worried about their older children and may feel guilty about their lack of time for them. They can feel lost and without an identity. Mothers also may struggle with emotional and perhaps physical space from their partner, such as sleeping in a different room to be with the baby. The mother who does not have a partner has additional challenges and logistics to work through. The sexual relationship is affected as well. Career, peer group, family, body, finances—no aspect of life goes unchanged.

Partners also experience adjustment after the birth, as they too have taken on a whole new role. They are experiencing their own transitions: career, concerns for older children, sexuality, a change in their primary relationship— all is in transition for this person, as well. They may also feel displaced. This new role or latest adaptation of the role is equally life changing.

Regardless of whether clients are partnered, regardless of their gender or sexuality, and regardless of any other factors, each situation is unique and requires an approach created by and specifically for those individuals. How can you support the family through this very normal and not always comfortable transition period? First is to see and hear each family member and let them guide you as to how you can support their unique experience.

Birth

The experience and outcome of the client's birth have a significant impact upon the responsibilities of the postpartum doula. If the mother has had a gentle, vaginal birth, her physical recovery will be easier than that of the woman who had a cesarean birth, significant episiotomy, or tear. Intervention or complications shape the weeks that follow. Breastfeeding may be harder after a long, medicated labor or a cesarean. Some doulas choose to specialize, offering either only birth or postpartum services. Even when specializing in postpartum support, it's important for us to explore and understand how birth is not just another day in a person's life (Simkin, 1991).

Our birth experiences shape how we see ourselves, our children, and our partners. Mothers who experienced a traumatic birth, to include obstetric violence, can experience challenging symptoms, to include PTSD (Simkin, 2019). While grateful for her healthy baby, a mother whose birth turned out differently from what she had wanted may have a maze of emotions to work through. She may feel sad, angry, hurt, frustrated, betrayed, or violated. Studies have shown that there is a connection between the experience and outcome of the birth and incidence of postpartum depression. It is not at all true that, "As long as mother and baby both come out of it okay (essentially, both surviving), everything is fine."

The postpartum doula listens to the mother. She's just had one of the most profound experiences of her life. If the mother chooses to share, it can be helpful for her to share her birth story in order to integrate her experience into her new identity. We listen to her story as often as she chooses to share it, and work to really hear her. There are bits of information here that will offer clues about what kinds of support may help. A helpful resource list to build is therapists who are versed in helping new parents process their birth experiences. Not all therapists will understand how pivotal this life event can be. Still others may understand the value but may lack a thorough understanding of the impact of interventions and the medical system as a whole. Helping parents to find the right person to walk with them through this process is of invaluable support.

The Birth Story—An Important Piece of the Puzzle

Birth leads us into the parenting experience to come. It shapes us, both physically and emotionally, for the rest of our lives (Simkin, 1991). It can impact long-term physical health, as well as subsequent pregnancies and births. Birth shapes how we see ourselves and our babies, as well as feelings about our birth support team. Birth itself brings the opportunity for healing of past losses through tender, uninterrupted, focused support. It can lead to self-empowerment; "I did that! I am amazing!" Just as easily, self-worth can plummet. A birthing mother can feel abandoned by her support team. She may feel judged as a failure. She may feel violated. The new mother brings this and any previous birth experiences into her time postpartum. Her own mother's birth experiences play into the emotional experience as well. Every mother marinades in her family's expectations of birth, recovery, and breastfeeding throughout her formative years. Those expectations may be represented by family members present at the birth, and they may be spoken aloud on an ongoing basis during the weeks and months postpartum if family members are present, either physically or emotionally. Suffice it to say, there are generations of shadow people present at every birth and postpartum experience. Remaining mindful of invisible influences upon her physical and emotional states will allow for a greater depth to the empathy and tenderness you bring to her care.

In addition to emotional adjustment, the physical aspects of labor and birth will have a direct impact upon physical recovery. Intravenuous (IV) fluids may lead to swelling in the mother and breastfeeding challenges (Kuwaja-Myles et al., 2015). Cesarean birth leaves mothers recovering from major abdominal surgery while also recovering from pregnancy and caring for one or more children. Tears and episiotomies cause pain and discomfort in positioning and movement. Not to mention that changes to the body brought on by labor and pregnancy themselves require weeks, months, and even years to recover from.

As the doula, modeling awareness of the birth experience, and patience in recovery and adjustment to the new self, is a tender gift. Honoring this portal to the parenting experience and giving it the attention that it deserves is a priority when doula-ing a family.

The Postpartum Worksheet

While the arrival of a new baby (or babies) is a time of great joy and excitement, parents may be unprepared for changes that lack of sleep, recovery from pregnancy and birth, and having an additional family member can have upon their lives and home. Unrealistic expectations derived from viewing family life through sitcoms and mainstream media can leave parents underprepared for life with their baby. They are under the mistaken impression that while they might need help for a week or two, things will then settle back into their regular lives—only now with a baby.

The reality is that the adjustment, both physical and emotional, lasts with some intensity for months following birth, and any parent of a baby or toddler will tell you that the changes do not end there. *The Postpartum Worksheet* is designed to help new parents have realistic expectations of their early months with a baby and set up their support network in advance.

Expectant and new parents will benefit for months from just a half hour's consideration of the following:

Support for Rest in the Early Days

During the days and early weeks following the birth of a baby, new parents need extra opportunities for sleep. Support during the night, naps, and tag-team parenting can all be effective sleep tools. In ideal situations, there is more than one adult (parent or not) available to meet the needs of the child(ren) at any given time so that turns can be taken, and naps or resting can happen. The goal is to schedule this type of support for several weeks—ideally, the first few months. Potential sources of help are family members, friends, doulas, and members of a worship community. When gaps are identified, take the time to strategize how to address this important need.

A Group of Friends Who are Also Parents of Young Babies

Common sense, life experience, and research confirm that having someone who can empathize with our experiences normalizes problems and makes them more bearable. These friends enhance rather than replace existing support networks. If several peers with young babies cannot be identified, strategize opportunities for building community. Find friends at childbirth education classes, prenatal/postnatal fitness classes, breastfeeding support groups, networking through friends, new parent programs, online discussion groups, and worship communities.

Nutritious Meals and Adequate Hydration are Very Important

While we are quick to encourage new parents to focus on healthy foods and staying well-hydrated, we are slower to facilitate that priority. It is unrealistic to expect new parents to meet this need themselves. Friends, family members, neighbors, coworkers, and worship communities can be a great support in this matter. It is advisable for parents to express what kinds of meals are preferred. Nutritious non-meals can also be requested, with a focus on foods that can be eaten with one hand—quartered sandwiches, trail mix, cubed cheese, and apple slices, so no parent goes without eating when there just isn't time to sit down for an official meal. Parents can plan ahead by double batching frozen meals, setting up an online meal train, and setting up delivery accounts with grocery delivery services in the months prior to the birth.

The Need for Knowledgeable, Empowering Breastfeeding Support

Breastfeeding is a natural process, but it does not always come naturally. Ideally, new or experienced parents are blessed with a community ready to provide education, screening, support, and guidance on breastfeeding. Appropriate support can help to avoid early challenges but often requires some planning.

Parents can consider who they have in their life who is not only emotionally supportive of breastfeeding (and this is crucial) but also is up-to-date informationally, can answer questions and make recommendations that will likely be helpful. Perhaps a coworker or friend experienced in breastfeeding, perhaps a family member. Even if that is the case (which hopefully it is), it would be wise to further prepare prenatally. This includes identifying local lactation consultants, doulas, and nursing groups. Have these names available in a list to include contact information, pricing, and other relevant details. Also helpful is to attend a breastfeeding support group several times while still pregnant. Watching babies nurse is normalizing, and so is hearing parents discussing their experiences. After the baby is born, the mother will be returning to a group rather than trying something new.

Support for Older Children

Older children will experience transitions of their own following the addition of a newborn to the family. Planning ahead for them to have time with their new sibling and also have special parent time is important. In anticipation of the birth, parents can consider what needs older children might have during the months postpartum. Are there specific times of day, rituals, or special activities that they want to protect? These should be planned for in advance. Also, it's ideal to consider the personalities of older children and strive for strategies that are a match for them when planning how they will weave this new person into the family.

Maintaining "Us" Time and Sense of Self–The Importance of *Me* and *We*

The addition of a baby to the family is a time of reinvention for parents. Every birth and new person added to the family includes transformation. Life has changed; never again will it be what it was. We have a new relationship in our lives and a new person to learn. Bodies change, availability to friends and activities change, and finances change. Our love that we were perhaps worried about dividing, in fact, doubles—or triples or quadruples.

For some people, the great swelling of love that they anticipated is slow to arrive, and this too is normal. There is so much going on for parents during the early parenting experience, and honoring this is a priority. Parents will benefit from planning for activities and breathers that help them to feel nurtured, rested, and energized. Some of these can be about each adult as an individual. Others can be about partnership and enjoyment of one another (when there is a partner). At times, circumstances may limit options to five minutes of peace for each adult to doze, meditate, walk, or practice gratitude. *We* time might simply be a snuggle, a shoulder, or foot rub that fits into a restful moment. Over time, creating opportunities to focus on the self as well as couple-ness remain priorities. Bringing these to the parents' attention prenatally may help them to remain mindful of their own needs.

Can we plan for every eventuality? No, but basic human needs such as food, sleep, and nurture are universal and will apply regardless of how things are going. The goal of this exercise is not to indulge in a fantasy of life with the baby; rather, the idea is to plan for life based upon realistic expectations.

Parenting Trends and Styles

Parenting styles vary among cultures, within faiths, socioeconomic structure, and location. Today, parents have access to similar information through the internet, publications, and television. Your clients will have goals for themselves as parents. These often include safety, nurture, and sleep. Parents also frequently worry about losing themselves or "getting my life back." While parents may have shared goals, there are different ways to attain them. At any given time, there will be trends in parenting; different schools of thought that purport that their own method is best for families. These range from *attachment* philosophies, encouraging breastfeeding, babywearing, and co-sleeping, to scheduled programs that are more *independence* focused. While some parents will completely subscribe to one school of thought or another, most eventually devise a style of parenting that suits their own family.

Choices can be difficult for new parents, as they may have people offering information from any or all of these schools of thought, insisting that their way is the best. The new parent, perhaps already doubting their abilities, can be overwhelmed. The doula can help by not pushing any one method. Our role is to provide information that is evidence-based. The doula ensures that the information they are offering is based on factual evidence rather than one person's opinion. Having offered information, make it clear to the parents that this is their family. They have the responsibility of care for this child, and they also have the privilege of making the choices that will nurture them through childhood.

No matter what the doula, mother-in-law, neighbors, or books may say, in the end, it is the parents who make the choices for their own family. The gift that the doula offers is being the person who encourages them to find the strength to make those choices. What feels right to them? Why does it feel right? Validate paths chosen. As parents feel supported in their decisions, they will develop confidence, and life as a family will feel more natural and easy.

While we don't tell our clients how to parent, it is acceptable to offer information from reliable sources that will help new parents in developing their parenting styles.

Helping Parents to Create a Peer Group

A powerful resource that we can offer new parents is friends. There is evidence that a supportive social structure can have a positive impact upon PMADs. Cronwett (1985) found that a vital skill for parents is the ability to augment their network of friends with a similar network of new parents. This is not to imply that older friendships should be dismissed. However, new parenting can be isolating, and building a peer group who are sharing similar life experiences can be of great benefit. Hearing other parents' stories can normalize experiences that may otherwise feel overwhelming and isolating, such as sleep deprivation and feelings of insecurity.

We, as the doula, can then offer them strategies for how to meet other parents. Whether spontaneously through walks to the park, online communities, or seeking out new parent classes and support groups, connecting parents with peers ensures the emotional support you are presently supplying will continue after your time together.

A tool that the doula can create for clients is an ongoing monthly calendar of opportunities for getting out and about. It may take an hour or so each month to create, but it is a long-lasting resource for your clients (and their friends as well, so it's a form of marketing). Try to fill each day with a support group, class, or experience that would be baby-friendly and offer opportunities to meet and share with other parents. Be sure that there are plenty of low and no-cost opportunities (popular parks or open museum days, for example), since we wouldn't want parents to remain isolated due to financial considerations.

Nourishing the Family

One of our goals is to nurture recovery and healing, and food plays a role in physical and emotional health. This is the case, whether or not you cook for your clients. If we are going to encourage parents to eat well, it is up to us to facilitate it. If not us, who are there specifically to help, who will? We need to walk the walk.

Help them to set up a plan if you have the opportunity to meet prenatally.

Preparing and freezing meals in advance is a great strategy. Taking friends up on offers and setting up a social support plan through an online option is a great start. Offer to sit with them and think through their needs and priorities.

Help them to have realistic expectations of life with a newborn.

Especially when there is only one parent (during the day or all the time), the opportunity to prepare a meal, sit, and leisurely enjoy it (not to mention clean up) may not present itself in the early months. Healthy grazing may be the "meal" for most of the day, sometimes even the whole day. Create a list of foods that can be eaten with one hand—cubed cheese, nuts, sliced apples, carrot sticks, quartered sandwiches—all of which can be prepared by yourself, other supportive adults, or the parents themselves. This way, they can be sure to eat every time the baby eats, a practice that is easy to remember.

Adjusting to life with a new baby can be emotionally challenging, and diet can help.

Basics, like remaining hydrated and keeping protein levels up, can help to keep mood level and help to flavor the adjustment experience (Ou & Greeven, 2016).

Offer practical help.

Help them to create grocery lists. Offer to go to the store and unpack the groceries. Sit with them as they set up online delivery accounts from local grocery stores. Find shortcuts. Don't just talk healthy lifestyle. Help them to live it.

Before you leave, make sure that fresh water and nutritious snacks are within reach.

This includes nights, since parenting is an around-the-clock role.

Dynamics of Partnerships

I'll state the obvious—not all partnerships consist of women/men or are female/male. Also, not all parents have partners. All individuals within all families are unique, and their preferences and challenges will express their individuality rather than their roles.

The purpose of this page is to state my intention for this writing to be inclusive and relatable. My own observation is that most relationship dynamics described in the pages to follow—the distribution of emotional work and the challenge of appreciating a partner's parenting style, for example, can happen in families of any makeup. While there are histories and complexities that are specific to LGBTQ+ families, there also exist universal joys and challenges.

Men and the role of father have their own histories and complexities, and these shape parenting expectations and experiences. These are also addressed in specific writings.

What defines a family? The family itself. Whatever words or identities they develop are what we, as their doulas, work with.

Families with One Parent

Another obvious point; some families are comprised of one adult and any number of children. Primary parents, grandparents, and others sometimes find themselves raising a child on their own (alone meaning without a partner in the home). The information listed here will be helpful in those situations as well.

Single parents face many of the same challenges as those with partners. Navigating the healthcare and childcare systems, financial challenges, and providing loving care to a child (or several) is quite a bit to take on. Doing so without a person to share ideas with, offer a break, and contribute to finances, can be all the more difficult. This also seems the appropriate place to acknowledge that having a partner does not guarantee any of the support listed above. Partners can bring quite a bit to the table, but the reality is that sometimes, they don't. It's not difficult to find new parents living in partnerships whose lack of support—or who only add to stressors—create circumstances that run parallel to those discussed here.

When we doula a family with one parent, considerations include:

✓ **Logistical.** Prior to the birth, what do they have and what do they need? Have they arranged their own meals for after the birth? Will someone help them bring the baby home from the birth center or hospital—a friend, a family member, or a doula? In these circumstances, it is more likely that the person doula-ing this family will be providing more logistical support than might be their norm.

✓ **Emotional.** Parents may feel that they are alone in the world with an enormous responsibility. At the same time, they may feel relief if they have recently ended an unhealthy relationship. Still, other single parents will have made a deliberate choice to have a child on their own. There may be insensitive questions asked about paternity and other comments made on parenting choices. Single mothers are sometimes concerned about being judged and stigmatized.

✓ **Financial.** While many things are the same as when there is a partner, it requires an extra layer of planning necessary when there is not a second person to serve as a financial net.

Specific suggestions for the support person:

✓ Remain nonjudgmental

✓ Plan ahead for meals

✓ Plan ahead for transportation

✓ Plan ahead organizationally

✓ While always a priority, here it is imperative to help clients build social support and access resources

✓ Anticipate needs

✓ Consider the need to be available off-hours when the parent needs someone to bounce things off of

As always, our role is to be NEAR—we nurture, educate, assess, and refer, often to the same resources as any other client. We may find a client on their own to rely more heavily upon the nurture aspect of our care if they aren't receiving that anywhere else in their lives. Similarly, we may have a focus on referring our clients, building community, and resources through the connections we help build.

(With thanks to Melissa Cook for sharing her expertise.)

All Parents are Parents

There is no one combination of people that means "family." Not all families include a father. This can be the case when there are two mothers. Or when a mother chooses to go through conception and/or pregnancy and parenthood on her own. Or when the father is separated from the family for legal or interpersonal reasons. That said, family dynamics often include a father. In some families, there are only fathers. The topic of fathering is challenging to tackle because of the diversity of possibilities. How to address, in primer-format, the enormity of validity and history that weave into every non-birth parent role? My approach has been to invite experts to address both the experiences of fathers and those of LGBTQ+ families in greater depth than I am qualified to explore.

While most people know that fathers have an important role in the lives of their children overall, many of us do not realize how profoundly their attitudes and actions can influence the postpartum experience of the entire family. Studies that don't include same-gendered partners can nonetheless provide information we can interpret and apply to any family. We know that support, to include peer/family support, has a profound impact on nursing. Along with emotional support and validation stands practical support, such as physical comfort, snacks, and the simple offering of a helping hand. In addition, we know that parents—regardless of gender—have an easier transition to new parenting within a network of friends who themselves have a new baby. A co-parent who is aware of this need, embraces it, and helps to build these relationships will be helping to compose a strong family unit.

Teaching parents concrete skills will help them to nurture their children. We can teach our clients infant capabilities and characteristics, so that they can know what to expect and get the most out of time with their baby. We can share evidence that approaches to parenting during the early days will have a marked effect on bonding in weeks to come. Many parents turn to bottle-feeding so that family members can help the mother and also feel the joy that comes with nurturing one's child. Instead of, or in addition to, the doula can facilitate nurturing skills. These include babywearing, supporting the mother with both words and actions while she nurses, and helping the mother develop a circle of social support that will guide them through the early months. All of these will make a difference in helping all parents to actively parent and support.

Another element to consider is how we are helping the mother, and the family as a whole, as they navigate the role of the co-parents. If our expectation is that their role is to 'help out' as in the past, we are doing everyone a disservice by disrespecting the competency of one parent while shifting the responsibility and workload principally upon the other. This attitude can lead to strain and resentment for both parents. That said, equal responsibility in parenting can require a paradigm shift. It can be a stretch for mothers to have confidence in the parenting intuition and skills of their partner. Some mothers confess to a philosophy of two approaches to an activity—*my way* and *wrong*. In this paradigm, partners experience frequent criticism and are challenged in developing their own parenting style.

A truly active parent takes on not just physical tasks but also the emotional labor of parenting (Hartley, 2018). Emotional labor can include the behind-the-scenes planning and remembering that enables the physical task to take place. Taking the baby to the pediatrician is one task. But who knew to make the appointment at a particular developmental age and made it? Who took time off? Remembered the appointment? Packed the diaper bag and made sure that the preschool-aged sibling would be picked up from school? This is the emotional labor behind a single activity. Active co-parents share in this aspect of life as well.

Becoming a Parent—A Metamorphosis

The journey into parenthood is a profound one. We go from child, sibling, and perhaps partner to a completely new role—that of parent. It is a time of great opportunity and great vulnerability. Expectations, and personal and societal histories, converge in the formation of a new and distinct entity with each and every child. Mindful of this transformation, our role is to meet the family with respect, patience, and trust in their innate abilities.

Where do the expectations of new parents come from? Experiences of:

✓ Any loss regarding their own parents

✓ The way that people they relate to have been treated as parents historically

✓ Observing their own parents' roles and experiences

✓ The role of parents within their community

✓ The role of parents within their culture of origin

✓ The role of parents within their partner's culture of origin

✓ The role of parents within popular culture

✓ Any absence of role models

✓ Observing the way others portray their experiences on social media

✓ Books they've read

✓ Classes they've taken

✓ Economic conditions

✓ Family leave policies

The transition to parenthood is all-encompassing. There is no aspect of life that remains unchanged. Identity, relationships, career, self-confidence, and sexuality—everything we can think of is affected.

Some parents lay eyes on their babies and fall in love. They seem to sail through the adjustment period. This is not everyone's experience, however. Parents sometimes take quite some time to fall in love with their babies, and this is also normal. It may take a while to bond, to lose the unspoken question, "When are this child's parents going to come and get them?"

The doula enters the picture at a time of great change. Hormone levels are rapidly changing. Parents are likely sleep deprived. Roles are shifting with a steep learning curve, requiring an entire set of skills for nurturing this baby. Self-confidence may initially be low, as the role of parent, or parent of this particular child, is new. It's not surprising that the doula needs to expect just about anything to happen. In this situation, it really could.

Self-confidence has a significant impact on a person's ability to approach any task, and parenting is no different. The doula can teach parents concepts and skills that will improve their skills in bonding with their babies. It is important to note here that "teaching" in the context of doula support likely will not include books or instructions. Educating is a broad concept, with many approaches. Often, we can educate through modeling with our own behavior, like washing our hands, wearing the baby while we prepare lunch, or our choice of words in encouraging still-young older siblings to use a gentle touch. Noticing aloud when we ourselves make a mistake ("I didn't fasten that diaper carefully—that would have made a mess!") can help to establish that none of us are perfect.

A calm baby who is growing appropriately will help parents to feel more confident in their skills. The doula can facilitate this by helping parents to use developmentally appropriate feeding techniques. Similarly, the doula can teach the value of skin-to-skin contact and babywearing. Babies nurtured in this manner grow faster and are more content, with less crying and fussing. Skills such as these can help parents develop confidence. As the baby grows and thrives, self-confidence will occur on its own.

The Myth of "Getting Back to Myself"

"Getting back to yourself" is a common topic of perinatal conversation. You can find it in chapters of books, in magazines, and in conversations. Getting your body back. Getting your life back. It sounds like it should be a top priority; after all, making ourselves a priority is a valid goal. There's a problem, though. There is no such thing. It's a misnomer. Something of a societal lie, because there is no going back. What new parents (and all the rest of us) are striving for is to become acquainted and comfortable with the person they now are. None of us can become the person we were before a physical event or a major life experience. None of us can become younger, or un-live what life has taught us.

This is not to imply that the situation is hopeless. Parents can strive for healthy, nourished bodies that are strong and fit. Parents can work toward career and life goals, and self-fulfillment. They can shoot for whatever stars their gaze fixes upon. The point here is that those things will happen as the people they are now and are becoming. Those pre-parent people? They're in the past.

The Basics of Nurturing Parents

✓ Listen.

✓ Cushion them and the baby. Give them permission and the ability to rest, eat, and care for nothing but themselves and their baby.

✓ Don't expect their transition to be smooth. Adjustment is different for each parent, with each baby, and at each developmental stage.

✓ Make it clear that they do not need to be able to do everything at once.

✓ Help them to follow their instincts. Affirm and honor the choices that they make.

✓ Help them to build skills in feeding and nurturing their baby so that they can build their own self-confidence.

✓ Help them to learn what to expect from a newborn, so they can provide appropriate care and experience successful interactions.

✓ Help them to enlist the support of peers to ease the adjustment into parenthood.

✓ Teach them babywearing so they can meet more than one person's needs at a time.

✓ Offer them timely referrals.

✓ Do everything you can to foster self-confidence.

✓ Remove your own agenda.

✓ Be sure that your support remains nonjudgmental.

Smooth Transition vs. Challenges

What might we observe when things are going smoothly?

✓ Some crying

✓ Exhaustion

✓ Interpersonal challenges (some bickering, for example)

✓ Some anxiety/hypervigilance

Here's where it can get tricky.

What might we observe when things are not going smoothly? When there are challenges?

✓ Some crying

✓ Exhaustion

✓ Interpersonal challenges (some bickering, for example)

✓ Some anxiety/hypervigilance

The challenge, then, is to somehow tease these apart. Preparation to work as a doula should include in-depth reading and exploration of numerous topics, to include PMADs (postpartum mood and anxiety disorders). One thing we know is that while all of the above experiences can be common, when adjustment is challenging, they are all bigger, faster, stronger—more crying, exhaustion to the point of not being able to sleep or not being able to wake, hypervigilance to an extreme extent (for example, parents can't sleep because they need to make sure that the baby is breathing) and symptoms that don't abate after a few weeks. In fact, they often increase.

When Adjustment to Life with a New Baby is Hard—What Do We Call It?

Really, what should we call it? Postpartum Depression? Perinatal Mental Health Challenges? PMADs (perinatal mood and anxiety disorders)? The colloquial "postpartum?" Does it matter?

For doulas, maybe it's better that we not call *it* anything but the behaviors that we've observed. The titles listed above exist for the purposes of insurance, research, and prescribing medication, but they serve very little use in everyday life. Since our roles do not include research, prescriptions, or the others, there is no reason for us to label our clients. In fact, it falls outside of our role.

Sometimes doulas use technical terms as a way of expressing their familiarity with the clinical world, part of our generalist nature. In this case, as with all others, we would do well to remain mindful of our non-clinical roles. Words are powerful, whether used on ourselves or others. Leave the diagnosing to the specialists. Our role is in providing the framework of support to help this family climb out of their low-point and begin to experience more pleasure. There is so much we can help with that the specialists will not be able to impact—we all have our own areas of support and expertise. For practical purposes, describing the present experience as hard and citing examples should be all that we need.

Perinatal Mental Health

Perinatal mood and anxiety disorders, commonly labeled as postpartum depression or just "postpartum," threaten the lives of women and their children, as well as the general health and emotional wellbeing of families. Although it is now in the public's eye, this experience is often undiagnosed, undertreated, and almost always under-supported. It is important to note here that the spectrum of postpartum mood disorders is quite diverse. PMADs frequently include high levels of anxiety, for example. While postpartum depression is a common PMAD, and it is the phrase that we hear the most, keep in mind that any number of behaviors can fall under this umbrella.

As doulas, our fears may have us focused on the most dramatic experiences we can imagine, perhaps involving the death of a mother, baby, or both. While these do happen, their instances are rare, thankfully.

More commonly, the joyous element of having a new baby in the home is disrupted. Most parents experience stress, sleep deprivation, and readjustment of their roles at some point after the birth of a child, but life feels mangeable, and pleasure is possible. When a parent is experiencing a PMAD, it may feel like all they experience are the hard parts. The mother may find that she can't relax and is worried all the time. She may find it very difficult to wake up and find herself without energy. On the other hand, she may find it difficult to sleep, even when the baby sleeps. She may cry quite a bit or feel numb. She may have difficulty bonding with the baby and find the child difficult to consider her own. Hypervigilance may make itself known through observations of compulsive diaper changing or overuse of hand sanitizers. Any of these are a hard way to live. As the doula, we can make a difference.

The Experience of the Partner in Perinatal Mental Health

It is important to mention that perinatal mental health challenges are not limited to birthing mothers. Partners, experiencing adjustment, stressors, and sleep disruption themselves, may also be in need of support and perhaps care to get through a challenging time. For this reason, *the partner* in this section could be any parent.

We know that when one parent is struggling, it colors the experience of the entire family. After months, or maybe years, of waiting for this baby, suddenly life turns upside down. The person they love may seem very different. The life they had imagined and planned now seems like a fantasy. They may find themselves responsible for almost everything that the family requires: cooking, cleaning, food shopping, laundry, even staying home from work for months to care for both children and co-parent. They may be at a real loss as to what has happened and how to proceed. The whole family needs help.

We can help the family at this time by educating the partner and recommending resources for them to learn more. The doula can teach the art of support to anyone in the home. A mistake that is frequently made is in telling someone that they "should be more supportive." This doesn't help. How should they be supportive? What can they do? What should they avoid? Clarifying the support role can ease worries and increase successes.

Both partners are going through a time of transition and may not be able to offer all of the support that their co-parent needs. The doula can make a difference here by offering direct support. Ask them specifically what they need. Do this prenatally whenever possible to set the baseline that everyone's needs are important. Often, the answer will be "just a little time alone, just a little space."

The doula can be a part of that transition time. We can support one parent and the children while the partner gets their bearings. We have the opportunity to provide hands-on education through modeling of behavior and attitude. The doula can encourage the partner to hold the baby skin-to-skin and become comfortable and close with their child. When more than one person supplies nurture to the child(ren), the primary caregiver, often the mother, can work on the self-care, rest, and seeking the support needed to heal.

Understand that the more one parent is struggling, the greater the burden upon their partner is likely to feel. If a Postpartum Worksheet, as described earlier, is not already in place, this is the time to sit down with whichever parents are available and create one. If one is already in existence, one of our priorities is to ensure that it is being put into effect.

How We Doula New Parents—No Matter How Things Are Going

There are things we know contribute to emotional wellness, choices and actions that are nurturing and productive, whether employed as a part of a positive plan for recovery from pregnancy and birth, or during times when the situation is more challenging.

In reading about how to support families experiencing a perinatal mental health concern, non-clinical suggestions for coping and recovery look a great deal like doula support—our support role with our clients remains the same, even when things are more challenging. Remember our acronym NEAR: Nurture, Educate, Assess, and Refer. What does this look like as we doula new families?

✓ **Nurture**

We nurture the body, with nourishing food and fresh water throughout the day. We nurture the body through touch, whether our own (only if invited, of course), perhaps with a foot or shoulder rub, or encouraging support people to offer touch. The goal is unlocking the love hormones, so it's not only those associated with stress coursing through the body.

We nurture through improved sleep, offering opportunities for naps, rest, and meditation when sleep is elusive, and teaching skills for when we are not there. Natural light, movement, and exercise as appropriate all help with recovery, and contribute to health in all people, regardless of age, gender, and new-parent status. While they aren't necessarily the cure, they can make a tremendous difference in some, and are always helpful, even when medical intervention is also necessary.

We nurture the emotional side of the person with our presence, willingness to listen, and acceptance of that person, wherever they are at that moment. We nurture with our belief that they are the right parent for this baby, that the answers will come to them, and the assurance that we will support them, along with others, until they do, and after. We nurture them by listening to their birth story without correction or adding our own emotions. We listen, and then we listen without minimizing, telling our own story, or encouraging them to feel differently from how they do.

✓ Educate

To begin, we educate new parents on how the care they take of their bodies, described above, will nourish their minds as well. Educate on realistic expectations of life with a baby, even when it isn't their first. We offer information on infant characteristics, care, and feeding to maximize the likelihood that things will go smoothly with a baby whose needs are being met. We suggest strategies for meeting the needs of older children to ensure a calmer transition.

✓ Assess

Our non-clinical assessment of the families we are with is ongoing, as it is throughout our everyday lives. When we doula a family, assessment is noticing. We notice when people are crying, more or less. We notice their affect—are they flat and seemingly numb? Joyful? Afraid? We notice their interactions with other family members, to include the new baby. We notice whether they are eating, when they seem sleepless, and everything in-between. We notice hypervigilance. We notice apathy. We observe their transition and draw upon our training and experience, considering how things are going and areas where we or others could help. Here is where the gift of doula-ing a family, rather than having a particular agenda (such as breastfeeding or clinical assessment), pays off. Our role begins with observation. We can make non-judgmental observations and suggest action in any area, from "There are so many visitors, so I just put a roll of paper towels in the bathroom for hand-drying," to "It's impossible to get all the sleep you need at night. Let me take the baby and toddler on a walk, and you just rest. That's why I'm here!"

✓ Refer

While we may know quite a bit, we still can't (and shouldn't aspire to) be experts in everything. Trying to be everything is not our goal. We seek to foster independence, to eventually make ourselves unnecessary. This can only happen by helping parents build skills, support, and systems that will work for them as they move forward. One of the best aspects of doula support is the referrals that we can offer to our clients, and we should be constantly building our list of offerings as well as being prepared to quickly network and investigate resources as needed.

Resources specific to postpartum emotional transition includes therapists and psychiatrists who specialize in PMADs. This seems simple but working through the quagmire of insurance and availability is sufficiently challenging on its own. Sprinkle in geography, transportation, finances, breastfeeding supportive (as appropriate), and seeking a match, and this aspect of things can be the very hardest to navigate while also being the most pressing.

Parents may also benefit from additional specialists, such as naturopaths, herbalists, homeopaths, and more. These are ideal practitioners to have on your resource list. Your resource list will also allow your client to have the best possible treatment should they choose one.

What Can I Do When Things are Hard?

Short answer: The same thing

Longer answer:

The most important thing you can do is to remain mindful of your role. When you are a doula or doula-ing a family, you are a layperson. It is not up to you to diagnose a condition, and it is certainly not appropriate for you to do so. It's not up to you to treat or cure anything either.

Why is this challenging? As the doula, you are a non-family member sharing their personal space and are privy to the intimacies of the life of this family. You are likely spending quite a bit of time with them. You experience their lives at home and are there for long enough that the masks we all wear slip and sometimes even shatter. As the doula, you will see, and perhaps feel, the pain, frustration, tears, and arguments. You may experience a parent who is despondent and does not respond to their baby's needs—cries and coos alike elicit no response. You may be supporting a mother who hasn't slept since the birth. You may be the person watching a family fall apart as one parent becomes less and less functional while the other (if there is one) takes on more of the burden, or doesn't, or perhaps spirals downward alongside them.

So, there you are, likely the person most prepared in this area who is supporting this family in their home, and I'm suggesting you not diagnose them. This may feel frustrating and limiting. I'll explain:

First and foremost, professionals who diagnose are licensed and have committed their careers to the education and expertise on the diagnoses themselves. So legally, it's not our role to tell someone, "I think you have postpartum depression."

That said, as the support person in the home, it feels like we are steeping in the experiences and emotions experienced within it. As doulas, we are trained in normal adjustment following the birth of a baby. We understand these things are never without challenges and can distinguish between typical ones (occasional crying in the early weeks, for example) and the scenarios described above. So, when we find ourselves in situations that fall outside of normal adjustment, what are appropriate steps to take?

Take off your cape.

Your role is to support, not to save. Unrealistic expectations of self as savior can create pressure in both yourself and your clients.

Stay within your role.

Nurture the heck out of them. Listen. Resource. Resource a lot.

Don't identify.

Perhaps you have a history of depression. Perhaps your story got really hard before it got better. Perhaps this situation holds some parallels—it's still not your story. You've never been this person, in this situation. Allow them the opportunity to forge their own path. Don't build your own expectations; if you do, your words and actions will betray you.

Avoid sharing your story.

People tend to struggle with this one, but there's a good reason to avoid it. First, sharing your story turns the focus toward yourself rather than the client. Next, your story can be frightening to others, who hadn't even considered that things could get as bad as you're describing them, even when that wasn't your intention in sharing. Also, the choices you made may not be the choices they'll make, and the baggage of fear of judgment will be sitting between you as time goes on. If at some point, you do feel compelled to share your history, keep it simple and without detail. Something along the lines of,

"I experienced significant anxiety after my baby was born. It took time and work, but now here I am," can establish your support as a peer. Of course, then you are opening yourself up to follow-up questions and all of the fallout above, so carefully consider even this.

Don't catastrophize.

This means don't build it up in your mind and make things worse than they are. Don't anticipate how bad things can get. Yes, things are challenging for this family—and therefore, for you—but things usually do get better, and this family has you. Believe in them.

Be prepared to take steps that may be outside of what other clients require while remaining mindful of professional and personal boundaries.

For example, while you might generally offer clients a printed or online monthly schedule of groups and other early parenting events they might want to attend, this client might need you to attend a group or two alongside her, so it feels more manageable. You may find yourself more involved, which can be appropriate in some situations. Be sure to keep checking in with yourself and make certain that any extra steps you're taking sit right with you. Compromising yourself will not serve your clients, because at some point you'll be exhausted or feel taken advantage of. Don't lose yourself as an ongoing priority.

Be aware of all family members, not just the mother.

Perinatal mental health challenges impact the entire family; everyone can benefit from an extra set of eyes and a sympathetic ear.

If the mother is despondent and the baby is not receiving much touch, seek workarounds: encourage partners to wear the baby and offer skin-to-skin time.

Grandparents and friends can participate as well, with the parents' permission. Sometimes a mother who is otherwise despondent is comfortable wearing the baby as more of an accessory, minus the eye contact. If this is the case, the baby is still hearing her voice and reaping many of the other benefits of being close.

Avoid private meetings of concern with other family members or friends, which will erode your client's trust in you.

Find ways to reduce your own stress. Bringing a fresh, open-minded presence to the home will serve you all well. If you come to a point when you feel the need to share concerns, do so openly and intentionally.

Additional Baby = New Family, First or Fifth

No matter whether it's the first or fifth, every new baby means a reconfiguration of the family and adjustment for all. Dynamics shift when an only child gains a sibling, when the youngest becomes the big sister or brother, and when parents are outnumbered—one parent has two children, or two parents have three. While experienced parents have a bank of knowledge to borrow from in terms of infant care and soothing, hindsight clues them as to what *didn't* work for them as much as what did. For this reason, they are often receptive to suggestions on self-care and infant soothing and feeding. They've never cared for this particular newborn before, with a temperament and biological structure all their own—which can mean different sleep and feeding experiences than they've experienced in the past. The addition of a newborn to a family with existing children requires an additional skill set—how to weave the needs and experience of this new person into existing dynamics and time-constraints.

Preparing Older Siblings

Parents sometimes find that the hardest part of preparing for their second, third, or even fifth born is anticipating the adjustment that older children will experience. Many are relieved to find that steps can be taken before the baby is born that will help to ease the transition for everyone.

The key is realistic expectations of and for everyone, including:

Do the older children know what newborns are like?

What they can and cannot do? Sometimes older children expect their new sibling to crawl or babble, and are disappointed when the baby does not. Big brothers and sisters have even been known to feed the baby finger food like Cheerios. Preparing older children well in advance will help with expectations. Weekly trips to the library and internet searches will provide age-appropriate materials. Simply spending time with friends or family with new babies is the most practical approach. This applies to all siblings to be, even those who are just a year or so old themselves.

While still pregnant, parents can set up friends, family, and childcare providers to come and visit after the baby is born. If the children don't know these helpers well, arranging time together so they don't feel they are left with strangers once the baby comes can make a difference. Parents can take some time to write down some basics on each child—what helps them fall asleep or when they're sad, favorite foods, and foods to avoid. These pointers can make a big difference for both children and caregivers.

It is helpful to identify rituals and activities with older children that are top priorities and plan around them. Babywearing and evening helpers tend to be efficient in these respects, as rituals are often baths and bedtimes.

As doulas, we can help parents to understand that their older child, who will soon seem so grown to them, is still a little growing person deserving of nurture. Just like parents, their lives are also completely changed, and it's not surprising if resentment or other feelings crop up. With a first baby, parents sometimes hold their child in their arms for the whole day. The same strategy can cause a lack of mobility and frustration when there are older children. Help them to feed the baby, tuck them in a carrier, and move on with the day, allowing the baby and older children both to feel nurtured.

Careful consideration of transitions like crib to bed, potty training, and weaning is advisable in the months before a new baby arrives. Remaining mindful that children sometimes regress after the addition of a sibling, parents can consider which transitions are imperatives and which might wait for some time after the birth. It's helpful if priority transitions take place well before the final weeks of pregnancy.

Newborn Capabilities and Characteristics

While we may not meet the family for hours, days, or even weeks following the birth, the doula's knowledge of newborn characteristics and capabilities can assist the parents in getting to know their baby and meeting their needs appropriately.

In years past, many people believed that newborns were almost completely undeveloped. They were thought to be largely impervious to pain, completely dependent, and non-interactive. It is challenging to discover that some parents and even some healthcare professionals today have much the same belief. There has been a wealth of research on the subject of the newborn, and thanks to the efforts of pioneers such as Brazelton, Nugent, Kennell, Field, Klaus, and Klaus, we have evidence proving that infants are far from little lumps.

Make it a priority to learn about newborns, their capabilities, and potential. Read, watch videos, take classes—learn all you can on the subject. Your understanding of the newborn will impact the care you provide—which, in turn, will impact the care infants receive from their parents.

Just to pique your interest, here are a few characteristics of newborns that you may not know:

✓ Babies are fascinated by the human face and can distinguish between scrambled and unscrambled images.

✓ Newborns can see most clearly at a range of eight to ten inches: about the distance from breast to the mother's face.

✓ Newborns can recognize familiar voices and sounds, including sounds heard in utero.

✓ Newborns prefer high-pitched voices and prefer that of their mothers above all others.

✓ Within a short time, an infant will prefer their father's voice above those of other men.

✓ Newborns respond to massage and touch with improved growth and a calmer demeanor.

✓ Newborn body movements often occur in rhythm with an adult's speech.

✓ A baby held skin-to-skin on their parent's chest, covered by a light blanket maintains their body temperature, and has better growth and increased oxygenation.

✓ A newborn will imitate the facial expressions of an adult who patiently and slowly models the motions (Klaus & Klaus, 1995).

A doula who understands newborn capabilities can foster parent/child interactions, leading to improved bonding and self-confidence. One challenge in parenting an infant is what can feel like a one-sidedness of interactions. Parents may feel that all of their energy is going into feeding, holding, and caring for this tiny person and that they aren't receiving much in the way of a reward. Parents are eager to interact with their baby and sometimes are anxious to get through early infancy so that they will be able to "talk" with their baby and get to know them better. Educating on where their infant is developmentally and how to communicate with them right now can help them to appreciate life today, rather than rushing through the early months.

New parents and the people supporting them may not realize the potential that exists for interaction beginning just moments after birth. When their babies smile, parents force themselves to dismiss it as "just gas," when, in fact, babies are primed for social smiles and interactions from birth. The doula can introduce the parents to their baby through modeling such interactions. When the doula observes aloud the baby mimicking sound or facial expression, parents will understand and internalize that their baby is already interacting with them. The excitement when a parent realizes that there is genuine communication going on with their baby is a moment they will remember forever.

Another way the doula can facilitate this process is to encourage the parents to hold and wear their baby as much as possible. As much as the doula, grandmother, or friend may love babies and ache to hold them, babies belong with their parents. It is tempting to offer to hold the baby for long periods of time so that parents can get a break, and this can indeed be helpful upon occasion to facilitate basic needs and rest. As an ongoing strategy, however, this amounts to putting a Band-Aid on a long-term reality. Parents do need a bit of space during the postpartum weeks. More importantly, they need skills that will lead them toward independence in caring for and interacting with their baby.

Parents who wear their babies will experience their greater contentment. They also have increased mobility for caring for and playing with older children and performing household tasks. After the initial "cushioning" period, the parents will assume a normal lifestyle, along with the responsibilities that it requires. If their support comes only in the form of infant care, the transition will be more difficult. The support person who helps new parents to wear their babies as both a coping and bonding strategy is offering them a step toward independence.

Also important are the six stages of consciousness experienced by newborns. The seemingly random movements of newborns actually fall into patterns. Each pattern holds potential for different types of interactions. Parents who understand these different states will have more successful communication with their infants. Just as adults are open to different activities such as playing and learning at different times, so are infants. Pay attention during your time with babies, and you will see how this information can help you to answer the baby's needs for stimulation, soothing, and even privacy for sleep. Babies communicate their needs and preferences quite clearly when we approach interactions from a two-sided perspective. Helping parents to develop these skills can provide valuable clues in the mystery of how to meet the needs of this new little person.

A tool that I gained during my NBAS (Newborn Behavioral Assessment Scale) training with Kevin Nugent at the Brazelton Institute is that of communicating with the parents through exploration of the baby. Not every client is comfortable opening up with someone they aren't already close with. Asking the parents to act as a guide to help you learn the baby offers so many positives. First, it establishes the parents as the experts, which, of course, they are. My heart melts every time I hear the parent of a two or three-day-old baby begin a sentence with, "He always..." It makes it clear that they are immersed in their bonding experience. We never start sentences about strangers with, "He always..." Once hearts are opened by sharing a moment as intimate as introducing their child, parents may begin to share further. Whether they do or not, it's a magical exchange every time.

When the Baby Cries—Strategies and Suggestions

Babies cry. It is among their primary means of communication and is a mechanism that ensures their needs are met; parents, therefore, need to be prepared for this challenging experience. In many Western cultures, however, there is perhaps an over-comfort with crying.

Yes, babies cry, but this doesn't mean that they *should* cry with any regularity or for an extended period of time. Crying is stressful for babies, parents, and anyone else within earshot. Unfortunately, childrearing practices of decades past combined with socialization by sitcoms create an expectation that crying is normal and to be expected. Most upsetting is the commonly received message: don't worry, they grow out of it.

For the baby and parent who are living with extended crying, a day lasts a week, and a week a month. These families can test the skills and knowledge of the doula, who, immersed in life with this family, is strongly motivated to help them find some relief.

As an unbiased support person in the home, the doula can sometimes offer unique insights within these situations. Doulas should ask themselves:

✓ Do we know why the baby is crying?

✓ Has a pediatrician or other clinical care provider been consulted?

✓ Has the clinical care provider provided a diagnosis and treatment plan?

Once it has been determined that there is not an obvious diagnosable condition, the doula can help the parents to explore, together with their care provider, other possibilities.

✓ Could it be feeding related? If weight gain is not optimal or the baby is having digestive problems, a lactation professional working in conjunction with the pediatrician may offer helpful insight.

✓ Is there a pattern to the behavior? Time of day, after eating, or something else? Are the feeding and care approaches being used appropriately with a newborn? Is the baby spending enough time skin-to-skin? Could the baby have physical trauma related to the birth?

✓ Is there a chance that a parent is anxious or depressed, outside of the obvious stressor of the crying?

While the doula is not qualified to diagnose or treat problems, we have the unique perspective of immersion in the home and everyday life of the family. It is possible that with a team approach and remaining mindful of scope, the doula can help parents to explore resources and strategies to relieve the situation. Such situations are yet another example of the need to keep our resources plentiful and up to date, as many solutions will fall outside of our support role.

Honoring Feeding Choices

Often, the method of feeding feels obvious and goes smoothly. It can also be emotionally draining and contentious. Food is an intimate experience and choice for all of us, and infant feeding is no different. Many factors figure into the decision of feeding method: culture, upbringing, finances, work policies, biology, and birth experiences all come into play.

As the person to doula this family, we may have our own opinions on the ideal strategy for feeding this infant. We've lived our lives, had our experiences, took classes, and more. There is no benefit to offering our opinion on the matter, even if asked. The priority is offering information as they work through their own decision-making process, then supporting through our words and actions. Regardless of feeding methods, we doula them by ensuring that babies are fed in the safest and most nurturing manner possible. In order to accomplish this, we take the time to educate ourselves on evidence-based feeding practices and use a variety of media to share that information with our clients. Books, videos, and modeling are all helpful tools in ensuring safe and loving feeding for all babies.

Breastfeeding Families

Parents often choose a doula to facilitate having the smoothest possible start with feeding. Doulas can also address challenges, should they arise. For this reason, it's our responsibility to be ready to educate on basics, identify challenges, and refer when necessary. This stands apart from the doula's own experiences and choices in parenting.

Breastfeeding requires support. Support doesn't necessarily mean instruction; it can look like many different things. Freeing up time is support. So is believing in the mother and baby's ability to work things out. Snacks and beverages are support. Sometimes being quiet is support.

While it is a natural process, sometimes nursing does not come easily. In traditional societies where people live close to mothers, sisters, grandmothers, and others who they interact with every day, learning about breastfeeding is a lifelong process. By the time a mother has children of her own, nursing has been a part of her everyday life. When she's starting out, or when problems arise, the experienced eyes of family members will recognize a problem and have strategies to help. In many Western societies, women give birth in hospitals, where they are reassured that using a pacifier or a few ounces of formula won't hurt the process. They then take the baby home, perhaps never to see another person who can help them with their breastfeeding. This is one reason why so many women feel that they "fail" at breastfeeding. Often, there is no physical problem in the mother or in the baby. The failure is in the lack of support, beginning at the societal level.

Our role, then, is to be there for the nursing mother with our sympathetic ear, education, experience, non-clinical assessment skills, and referrals.

Supporting the Breastfeeding Family: Basics

✓ Have a strong, evidence-based foundation in how breastfeeding works.

✓ Teach clients about how the process works, prenatally, if possible.

✓ Be sure to use a teaching approach that is a match for their learning style.

✓ Observe the mother nursing and make recommendations that are within your scope.

✓ Know what is not within your scope. This is everything that is not within the realm of normal.

✓ Know who to refer a mother with breastfeeding concerns to.

✓ Constantly update your contacts so that you know that you're connecting her with the best possible resources. Do you know the lactation consultants in your area who come to the home? Take insurance? Work on a sliding scale or pro bono? The location and offerings of the local WIC office? What nursing mothers' groups are in the area?

✓ Educate her family members about how to support her.

✓ Help her to assess whether her pediatrician is supportive of breastfeeding.

✓ Help the mother to rest.

✓ Minimize responsibilities of organization, older childcare, and meal preparation to allow her to rest close by her baby, so cues can be quickly identified and needs met.

✓ Help the mother to eat and drink well so that she has energy.

✓ Support the partner (when applicable) and siblings of a breastfeeding baby.

✓ For clients who are both breast and bottle feeding, provide information on strategies that are more compatible with a smooth transition between the two, such as paced bottle-feeding.

Supporting Breastfeeding: Suggestions for Partners

✓ Assure the mother that her milk is the ideal food for their baby.

✓ Help her to be physically comfortable while nursing.

✓ Bring a snack and something to drink while she nurses.

✓ Do not assume that gas pains or a crying bout are related to the mother's milk. It puts pressure on the mother and also is not accurate.

✓ Use your visual perspective to help with positioning and latch.

✓ Encourage her to nurse on cue. Learn the cues.

✓ Watch the baby rather than the clock; both parents will get to know the baby better this way.

✓ Meet the needs of older children and pets so she can relax into her role.

✓ Develop skills for nurturing and soothing the baby, such as babywearing.

✓ Be patient. Remember that she and the baby have never done this together before. It often takes several weeks before breastfeeding begins to feel smooth.

✓ Ask for help when you need it.

Breastfeeding: The Importance of Referrals

When it comes to breastfeeding, the postpartum doula's role is to support. Unless the doula is also a lactation consultant, they are not an expert. The lactation professional assesses and creates a strategy, and the doula helps to execute that plan. The postpartum support community is at its most functional when each member of the support team conducts themselves within their professional boundaries. When in doubt, refer it out!

A lactation professional is not the only referral you should be prepared to offer your clients to support breastfeeding. Research indicates that peer support, such as that offered through La Leche League or other nursing mothers' groups helps to improve the likelihood of breastfeeding success (Olson & Haider, et al, 2000). Know what is available in the communities that you support, as well as the strengths and specialties of different groups. Not every group will suit the personality and needs of every mother.

The philosophy of the pediatrician, obstetrician, or midwife can also impact the nursing experience. One very simple assessment is to ask the practitioner to list a few of their favorite breastfeeding books and several local breastfeeding resources. If they aren't able to offer these, they may support breastfeeding with their words but have not taken the time yet to prepare themselves to fully support breastfeeding families. If the mother is planning to breastfeed and her practitioners are anything other than supportive, the doula can be prepared with names of practitioners who are breastfeeding-friendly.

As you can see, the doula needs to have much more to offer than the experience of perhaps having nursed their own children. Be sure to purchase quality books on breastfeeding, attend local and online classes on breastfeeding support, attend related conferences, and make it a point to continuously build your knowledge and skill in this area.

On the Support Needs of Families:
Other Voices

The Post-Baby Body—Awareness and Care

Years ago, in addressing challenges within my own post-body, I met Anne Duch, PT, and life changed for me—and for the many people I sent her way in the years that followed. At that point, I had four children and had been mothering for about 18 years. I was a birth professional, trained in pre- and postnatal fitness and childbirth education, as well as being a doula. I had a history with movement and exercise. All in all, pretty empowered, yet there was my body, experiencing challenges experienced by my mother and grandmothers before me. No worries; I was a doula, knew how to resource, and I lived in a different age. I found my way to Anne, and after minimal physical therapy visits and a whole lot of time and work on my own, my problems disappeared.

This is something women need to know, I (obviously) concluded, so I started asking Anne to come speak to my doula training and to the new-parent support groups that I facilitated. I hung upon her every word, as if my very well being hinged upon it—because it did. I wove Anne's observations into my doula practice and into every interaction I had with new and expectant parents. Even though I had worked in the field for years, her recommendations were cutting edge at the time, and for many, will still be received as a drastic departure from what they've been told by their community and even caregivers today. What we know now is that we, as birthing parents, can impact our own physical health through our choices and actions, empowering information for many. It's overwhelming information for some, who might feel uncomfortable with the prospect of taking responsibility for their own wellbeing. While many things are out of our hands, there are things that we know:

✓ **Our birth experience and interventions interpret into our post-birth bodies.**

Episiotomies, tears, and cesarean births all come with potential fallout for our bodies.

✓ **Birthing one or more children does not equate with a life of incontinence, ending with eventual surgery.**

✓ **Pain with sex is not normal and is often not the result of tension.**

The advice of "have a glass of wine and relax" is insulting because it minimizes an often real, physical problem that would be actually solved if it were acknowledged and addressed, rather than treated with wine.

✓ **Recovery from each birth takes time—way more time than we are led to or want to believe.**

We only have one opportunity to recover from each birth. After that, any reversal of challenges like incontinence and pain are work and are undoing the damage that was done when we didn't invest in ourselves and fully heal initially. I explain to clients, "I understand that 28-year-old you is feeling pretty good right now and ready to launch. Keep in mind that 50-year-old you is in there too. And 70-year-old you." The older "us" requires more healing time. Invest. Invest in your future wellness. Rest. Recover. Find the community and professionals you need. You only have this one chance.

Having added my voice, here are words from Anne. Please note that they are not to be taken for medical advice; not every option is available or best for every person. Birthing parents should consult their care provider about their postpartum recovery and seek out additional professional voices when their needs are not yet met.

Words from Anne Duch, MTP, WCS, RYT

One of the biggest challenges a woman faces during the postpartum period is the physical recovery from her delivery. This recovery is made more challenging by the accompanying sleep deprivation and emotional toll of navigating the new and ever-changing world of motherhood.

The mom will require both reassurance and guidance when it comes to her physical recovery. Gone are the days of telling her that leaking urine is just simply what happens after a woman has a baby or that pain with intercourse is now a fact of life. These two overused statements are just plain false and should be banished during any conversation with a woman who has just birthed a human.

✓ **Urinary leakage, difficulty holding back gas, and pain with intercourse are three examples of pelvic floor dysfunction that can be present in women who have had either a vaginal or a cesarean birth.**

> These situations are typically a result of the pelvic floor muscles being incredibly overactive, measurably weak, or simply uncoordinated within the core muscle system.

✓ **Women who have had a C-birth will benefit from some discussion about mobilizing their incision site.**

> This may include desensitizing the incision by rubbing it gently with a cotton ball or soft material during the first couple of weeks postpartum. The same type of scar mobilization can be utilized in any area within the pelvic floor where tearing or an episiotomy was performed.

✓ **The mother should be encouraged to begin belly or ribcage breathing the day after the baby arrives.**

> This type of breath, where she works on allowing the belly and ribcage to expand on the inhale and gently draw down and in on the exhale, optimizes pressure management of the abdominal cavity, lessening

the pressure being exerted on the bladder or bowels internally. It also promotes abdominal muscle activation, which is helpful following several months of the belly muscles being on a stretch.

✓ **During the first 7-10 days post-vaginal delivery, management of pelvic floor swelling is important.**

This is a perfect time to begin to practice very gentle Kegel contractions. In doing so, advise the mom to gently lift the muscles between her pubic joint and her tailbone, followed by a gentle letting go of those muscles. Some women will have a better connection to the activation of the pelvic floor muscles (a Kegel) by imagining a closing of the vaginal opening. Of equal importance when cueing Kegel contractions is to advise the woman to then let go completely afterward. It is the *excursion* of the Kegel—the lift **and** the lower—that is of importance, not necessarily just the strength of the contraction.

As Mom starts to be able to feel the lift and lower of the pelvic floor muscles, she should start to link them to her breath. She will inhale through her nose, allowing her belly and ribcage to fill with breath. This will be followed by an exhale through her nose, noticing her ribcage and belly drawing down and in, while performing a lifting up/closing of her pelvic floor muscles. As she cycles through her breath, she will continue to release the pelvic floor muscles on the inhalation and draw them up and in on the exhalation. This can be an exercise in coordination. If it becomes too complicated, scale back to working on one thing at a time—breath first, Kegel contractions second.

✓ **As the new mom makes her way through the first 4-6 weeks postpartum, she will start to become more active and may be anxious to get back to whatever form of exercise she did prior to having her baby.**

Encourage her to use those 4-6 weeks to heal completely, eat well, and rest as much as possible.

✓ **Upon having her 6-week postpartum check-up, Mom is often told everything looks great "down there" and that she is ready to get back to exercise and cleared for resumption of intercourse.**

> In actuality, the 6-week check-up is simply a measure of soft-tissue healing, which in the absence of infection or some other complication, takes place during a 4-6 week window in a healthy individual.

> Quite often, the new mom does not feel ready for intercourse at that point because she is nervous that it will hurt, or she is experiencing urinary leakage or trouble holding back gas. This is a perfect time for her to begin to assess herself both externally and internally while in the shower.

✓ **When the mom and partner are ready to engage in sexual activity, ensure them both that any pain with penetration is common but not normal.**

> It is also so incredibly treatable. The muscle spasms that are likely causing the pain can be released by a combination of internal work and appropriate hip exercises to address imbalances that often come with pregnancy. Refer them to a women's health physical therapist for further evaluation.

✓ **The same advice holds true for any woman who experiences loss of urine with coughing, sneezing, laughing, or position changes, as well as for those who are experiencing urgency.**

> It is common post-baby, but not normal. If it continues to happen 16-20 weeks postpartum, refer to a women's health physical therapist for specific recommendations. Each case is vastly different, but all are treatable in some way.

The work of Anne and others who focus on recovery significantly impact the quality of life experienced by new mothers. As the person to doula this mother, our contribution is being aware that these concepts and services exist and creating options by connecting the parents with what is available in their communities.

Understanding Dynamics of Oppression, Power, and Privilege When Supporting Families

by Naima Black

What do people mean when they categorize a group as "underserved?" Is this an adequate or appropriate term? Does it allow for a smoothing over of the depths of inequity our society continues to experience and perpetuate? The language of "service" may have some problematic elements in that it implies "a handout" solution and may continue cycles of condescending or patronizing behaviors. I would pose possible alternate language: *people who are poorly supported or not supported at all, people whose power has been stripped away.*

People, especially parenting people, who bear the heaviest burden of inequity in our country are predominantly black, brown, and poor. The challenges and barriers they face are largely a result of intersecting systems that are set up, both intentionally and unintentionally, to limit, minimize, criticize, and often criminalize their lived experience. Ongoing microaggressions that are at the core of racist behaviors and implicit bias are the status quo when people have to deal with systems and authorities tasked with providing assistance.

Lived experiences of poorly supported communities:

✓ **Living conditions**

> Violence in neighborhoods; over-policing of communities; high rates of incarceration; food deserts; extremely underfunded schools; unsafe and unkempt play/recreational spaces; crowded living spaces without privacy; isolated living situations.

✓ **Economics**

> Decreasing public assistance benefits; restrictive public assistance criteria, including difficult access to childcare and childcare subsidies; lack of a living wage; long work hours; difficulty making appointments and getting to them.

✓ **Health and wellness**

> Different standards of care (and/or perceptions thereof) for folks with Medicaid; who gets drug tested at childbirth and what happens as a result; limited options for laboring, childbirth place, and provider; almost non-existent 4th-trimester care.

Given that finally, there has emerged more mainstream acknowledgment of the deep and persisting harm that racism inflicts upon people of color in this country, particularly those who are descendants of enslaved people, it is beholden upon us all to engage in the hard work of undoing racism. Focusing on the band-aids and fixing symptoms is a fleeting solution and self-serving for those who need to feel they are doing some good.

In the meantime, what should we do and not do?

✓ Shift the narrative from "empowering women" to "stop taking women's power away," and acknowledging and stating that parents are the experts on their own babies.

✓ Advocating for expanded coverage of community doulas, birth, and postpartum with a focus on training people of color.

✓ Reducing the use of blame and patronization (i.e., safe sleep practices; how one chooses to feed their baby, etc.).

✓ Pushing for more home visiting CHW, Peer Counselor, and Nurse programs for parents and babies.

✓ Building a workforce sector with people who represent communities ethnically and linguistically, and who receive comprehensive training, including understanding and responding to trauma.

A few thoughts when working with families who have lived experiences of racism, poverty, trauma, and poor resources would be (these are things we should practice with everyone):

✓ **Assume each person knows their body, family, and community.**

✓ **Listen carefully and fully first (always listen more/talk less), then:**

> ✓ Acknowledge, affirm, praise, and encourage.
>
> ✓ Ask permission to offer your thoughts, targeted information, and resources before sharing them (this does not require you telling all of your stories that seem similar).
>
> ✓ Develop and work hard on being truly empathetic in body and language.
>
> ✓ Pay attention to who is present and the environment and show respect and interest (for example, if shoes are all lined up at the door, offer to take yours off).
>
> ✓ Let them know you are not the expert and if they have needs or questions that you can't address, admit it and offer to help them find what they need.

✓ **Don't try to make decisions for people or judge the decisions they make.**

✓ **Know that you can't fix other people's problems.**

✓ **Be curious and show interest in someone's culture if different than your own.**

✓ **Build trust, not walls (be genuine).**

✓ **Practice self-care.**

Supporting LGBTQ+ Families in the Postpartum Period

by Morgane Richardson

One day, we may look back on books about conception, pregnancy, and the postpartum period and shudder at how exclusionary they were. In 2019, people write of the postpartum period as though it only impacts cisgender moms and dads (cisgender is a term used for people whose experience of their gender agrees with the sex they were assigned at birth), and we continue to use language that assumes that all people who give birth or adopt are women/men or male/female. But we know that simply isn't the case. It never was, and it isn't today.

This section aims to open a conversation that many birth workers are trying to navigate; what is the experience of birth like for members of the LGBTQ+ community, and how can we (the partner, doula, grandmother, or best friend) support people who identify as LGBTQ+ and gender nonconforming in having a fourth trimester that is respectful, inclusive, and empowering. This section is by no means exhaustive; in truth, an entire book can and should be written about this topic. I also want to acknowledge that I am writing this section from my perspective as a queer, cisgender woman of color, and thus, there are certainly voices, experiences, and realities that are missing here. I don't know it all, but my hope is that you are provided with a tiny taste that inspires you to take steps—no, leaps—into exploring what it means to be an ally for LGBTQ+ people who are in the throes of creating their families.

On Using Gender-Inclusive Language

The terminology used in this section may roll off your tongue, or it may feel completely foreign. I recognize this might be the first time some readers are engaging with words like intersectionality and cisgender, and so I've made a point of including some crowdsourced definitions of terms at the end of the section.

I would like to acknowledge the use of the term LGBTQ+ here. I personally also struggle with the use of acronyms because they can be problematic and exclusionary. Acronyms can be useful, but they can also be dangerous in their desire to clump together a group of people who don't all share the same lived experiences. For the sake of this section, I've chosen to use LGBTQ+, as it is most commonly used in literature, but I acknowledge that it doesn't include all gender identities and sexual orientations.

Language is a reflection of the culture and society we live in; it has the ability to maintain or redesign that world. Language is a powerful social and political tool that can foster discrimination or empowerment. Can you say that you are an LGBTQ+ competent care provider if you memorize a few terms? Are you an ally the second you use "the right words" when supporting a family who identifies as LGBTQ+? Certainly not but becoming familiar with gender-neutral language, and using it within your life, is an important piece of being an LGBTQ+ ally.

While I have shared a few terms with you here, I encourage you to continue doing your own research. In growth comes discomfort, right? I encourage you to be uncomfortable; place yourself in situations and environments where you will be pushed to further explore these identities and concepts. I'll be there too.

Intersectionality: Not all LGBTQ+ Families Are the Same

I want to take a moment to mention the importance of intersectionality. Intersectionality, a term coined by Kimberlé Crenshaw in 1989, is a framework or theory that takes into account an individual or group of people's overlapping identities and experiences (race, class, gender identity, religion, sexual orientation, disability status, etc.) to understand the oppression they face.

Intersectionality acknowledges that we cannot examine one part of our identities separately from all the other parts. Furthermore, each one of our identity markers inform the others. While we are talking about queer or LGBTQ+ families, remember that each of these people has other identities and realities that intersect with their lives and impact their access to choice. A White, middle-class lesbian family may, in fact, experience parenting completely different than a family who identifies as a Black upper-class genderqueer.

Many of the postpartum needs for LGBTQ+ families will be the same as any other family; new families need guidance about the care of their newborns, emotional support, and words of encouragement, help around the house, and access to resources for lactation support, sleep, feeding the baby, and the like. That said, LGBTQ+ families don't all have access to the same resources, including access to queer-affirming care. Members of the LGBTQ+ community will experience differences in access to or availability of healthcare facilities and services according to social determinants such as culture, race, socioeconomic status, religion, country or region of residence, sex, gender, and sexual orientation.

While the needs of LGBTQ+ families may appear similar to the heterosexual, cisgendered, White family on the surface (help parent shower, feed baby, etc.), caretakers must also be aware of the social determinants of health that may prohibit a family from gaining access to important resources, including paying for a lactation consultant, postpartum doula, etc. Sometimes, the most important thing a friend, family member, or postpartum doula can do is acknowledge our limits, accept that a family may need more than what we can offer, and refer out to strong resources.

Before A Postpartum Doula Comes into the Picture

There are a variety of ways in which people and specifically, LGBTQ+ families, become parents. This can have an impact on the decisions families choose and sometimes must make for their perinatal care.

One big deciding factor is the financial investment of creating a family; the cost of conception can be high if one or more people in the family are choosing to carry a pregnancy. On average, a person will spend about $1800-$2000 each cycle of intrauterine insemination (IUI). This is for sperm, sperm shipping/storage, and at-home care provider services for basic IUI. In-vitro fertilization averages roughly $12,000 per cycle. This does not include consultation fees, medical fees (sonogram, testing, hormone injections, etc.), and is oftentimes not covered by insurance for LGBTQ+ people. The cost of surrogacy is, on average, $98k-$140k, and the costs of adoption vary between 0-$2,500 (via the foster care system), and $8,000-$40,000 (independent adoption).

While the hope is that every person who chooses the path to parenthood is surrounded by people who will provide them with support, the reality is that we still live in a highly homophobic society that doesn't always view LGBTQ+ families as, well, families. In this way, you might find that the family you are supporting is navigating shifting dynamics with their parents, grandparents, siblings, etc., as well as unwarranted, negative feedback from their communities regarding their decision to become parents.

Recommendations for the postpartum doula:

✓ **Ask questions on a need-to-know basis.**

> Don't ask people how they conceived unless it is medically necessary for you to know for their treatment. Imagine asking a heterosexual person or couple how they got pregnant!

✓ **Acknowledge that LGBTQ+ couples commonly have to spend additional money to conceive.**

Depending on their financial situation, they may or may not have the same flexibility to choose or have access to care for their postpartum.

✓ **Respect that there may have been a long (or short) emotional journey to get to the conception phase.**

Even if it was "easy," LGBTQ+ families may have had to navigate complicated family dynamics, the stress and long wait of building savings, and more to get to the point at which you're now meeting them.

Emotional Health

Providing support for emotional health is an incredibly important part of supporting clients in the perinatal period.

Unique challenges might include grandparents who do not recognize the new baby as part of the family; the lack of models of LGBTQ+ parenthood and new families; and acceptance or comfort among other new parents.

The path to parenthood can be seamless, or it can be difficult for LGBTQ+ families. It is important to recognize that all families come to parenting in different ways: planned for and unexpected, via surrogacy, domestic or international adoption, IUI, ICI, IVF, or sexual intercourse with their partner(s). While you may not be the one to provide the emotional space your friend, family member, or client needs as they go through the stages of these processes, you can ensure they have access to the support and resources they need as they expand their family.

Breast/Chestfeeding

There is a lot of pressure around feeding babies, both self-imposed and from the larger birth and parenting communities. When I took my Certified Breastfeeding Counselor training, I was told, "Only a small percentage of people can't physically breastfeed their babies. The main reason people think or feel they can't feed their children using their breast/chest is because they lack the resources and support to guide them through the ups and downs of breast/chestfeeding." Now imagine if the literature and images you saw of people feeding their babies didn't represent your family. Would you feel comfortable reaching out for help if you didn't see yourself reflected in the parent groups or books you were researching? Maybe, but maybe not.

The sad truth is, images of people feeding their babies are largely able-bodied, Caucasian women with medium-sized beige breasts. There exists very little research that expands lactation support to families who are LGBTQ+ and/or gender nonconforming. In fact, I did a Google search for "breastfeeding," and I had to scroll down a bit before I found a brown person feeding their baby. When I Googled breast/chestfeeding, the information was more sensationalized news headlines than helpful, evidence-based research.

I am a bisexual, cisgender woman of color who lactates, and at the time of writing this, I'm parenting an 8-month-old child with my wife. For me, figuring out how to feed our baby was more challenging than an unmedicated home birth. I'm forever grateful that I am a birth worker because I knew immediately where to reach out for support. More than that, I had a community of like-minded friends who understood my tears of frustration and the joy that comes with getting a baby to latch while in a carrier. And yet, every time I breastfed my child, whether it be at home or in public, I still feel as though I am making a political statement. "Look at me!" I think. "I'm a Black, queer woman, and that's right, I'm breastfeeding!"

My wife did not carry our daughter, and while she has zero desire to get pregnant and give birth, she wanted to breastfeed. She tried inducing lactation with herbs, acupuncture, and lots of dry nursing, and it was a disappointment when it didn't happen. While other queer families talked about the idea of inducing lactation for the non-gestational parent, we knew of no one who had taken the steps to do it. My wife did end up dry nursing our daughter for the first few months of her life, and despite having a large network of queer families in Brooklyn, NY, we don't know of many other people who openly speak about doing it themselves. Hopefully, we look back on these words in shock at how alone and how secretive we felt we had to be.

There are so few detailed research studies, books, or websites that walk you through the process of inducing lactation or that discuss the emotions that come up when navigating differing relationships to feeding babies within the queer community. So, how can you help as someone who is trying to be supportive of the LGBTQ+ person in your life who is expanding their family?

Recommendations for the postpartum doula:

✓ **Don't assume how a person is going to feed their baby/babies.**

It's possible that both parents, only one, or none physically can or will breastfeed. Instead, ask them, "How do you want or plan to feed your baby?"

✓ **Be mindful of the language that you use.**

Use terms like "feeding your baby" and chest/breastfeeding rather than assuming someone is breastfeeding.

✓ **Learn about a range of nursing options.**

Research what it means to induce lactation (the Newman-Goldfarb protocol) and be mindful that this is a major endeavor, not a fun quirk of queer parenting. Parents might also opt to use a supplemental nursing system, or simply to comfort or dry nurse without feeding/lactating.

✓ **Make sure to equip families with lactation consultants/counselors who are aware of the specific needs of LGBTQ+ families.**

Generate a list of care providers (lactation consultants, herbalists, etc.) in your area who are familiar with this in case you need to refer out.

✓ **Support the choices families make, whether or not they align with what you want.**

Create a supportive space for all family members to do skin-to-skin support in the postpartum, free from shame and discomfort.

Legal Rights and Obstacles

Unfortunately, not all family make-ups are recognized around the world. While a birth parent will have legal custody over a child, in LGBTQ+ relationship or marriage, the partner may not have legal rights. Families may or may not choose, or have the right, to go through a legal process to adopt their children. For those who are going through any type of adoption process (including second-parent adoption), they will likely need to prepare their residence for a home visit by a social worker, solicit written character referrals from friends and colleagues, and provide extensive financial and medical records.

Many people assume that a birth certificate confers parental rights over a child. It does not; birth certificates are simply a presumption of parentage and not recognized as absolute proof of parentage. Adoption law is the domain of courts and legislatures. In 2019 in the U.S., where I live, the DOMA (Defense of Marriage Act) ruling has no bearing on whether or not same-sex couples have the same legal parental rights as heterosexual couples. It is legally advisable for non-biological parents to get an adoption or parentage judgment to ensure that their parental rights are fully protected, no matter where they move or travel to, even if they are married, in a civil union, or a registered domestic partnership. However, each family will have to navigate the pros and cons of pursuing adoption. It is important to support the family in their choices.

Recommendations for the postpartum doula:

✓ **Respect that families may have to make postpartum decisions based on a social worker's home visit requirements for adoption purposes (i.e., co-sleeping vs. crib).**

✓ **Remember that LGBTQ+ families may be saving funds for legal fees, which can impact the choices they make about their care providers (ability to hire a lactation consultant, postpartum doula, etc.).**

✓ **Look into second-parent adoption laws.**

If your clients ask you, you then have the resources to be able to help them understand the breadth and limits of their rights, and whether there is a need to contact a lawyer to discuss their options.

Conclusion

During pregnancy, birth, and the postpartum period is not the time for families to teach others about the kind of healthcare support they want and need. They are reaching out to you for that support, which means that we, as friends, family, doulas, and healthcare providers, need to educate ourselves. Whether you are a doula, a medical care provider, or a mother-in-law looking to find ways to support your LGBTQ+ friends/family in this transition, here are some reminders:

✓ **Educate yourself.**

Read, research, and listen to the people who are experiencing the oppression and the challenges. This cannot be emphasized enough.

✓ **Know yourself and your limits.**

Get in touch with how you feel about the issues, yourself, and your comfort level with the pros and cons of being an ally. When you have reached your limits of knowledge or patience, help the person find the appropriate resources.

✓ **Create a comfortable setting.**

Be conscious of the things you use to decorate your work environment and the tools/resources you bring to your classes (i.e., childbirth education).

✓ **Confront jokes and slurs.**

Silence may communicate you're condoning oppressive statements.

✓ **Challenge your community and colleagues.**

Take every opportunity to share your information with them.

✓ **Know that each of us are the experts on our own experiences.**

✓ **Allies make mistakes.**

Apologize and learn from your experiences

Terminology

Ally: A person who is not a member of a targeted social group who takes action or speaks up to challenge discrimination or prejudice against a targeted social group.

LGBTQ+: An umbrella term referring collectively to people who identify as lesbian, gay, bisexual, transgender, questioning, and/or queer. Gay used to be the general phrase used, but now LGBTQ+ is the more current and inclusive term.

Lesbian: An identity for people who are female-identified and who are attracted sexually/erotically and emotionally to some other females.

Gay: An identity for people who are male-identified and who are attracted sexually/erotically and emotionally to some other males. Gay used to be an umbrella term to refer to all lesbian, gay, and bisexual people but the more inclusive term used now is LGBTQ+.

Bisexual: An identity for people who are sexually/erotically and emotionally attracted to some men and women.

Transgender or Trans*: A broad umbrella term used to describe people whose gender expression is nonconforming and/or whose gender identity is different from their sex assigned at birth. Transgender people may or may not choose to alter their bodies hormonally and/or surgically. People must self-identify as transgender in order for the term to be appropriately used to describe them.

Queer: An umbrella term used to describe a sexual orientation and/or gender identity or gender expression that does not conform to heteronormative society. While it is used as a neutral, even positive term among many

LGBTQ+ people today, historically, it has been negative and can still be considered derogatory by some.

Cisgender (or cis): Describes related types of gender identity where individuals' experiences of their own gender match the sex they were assigned at birth.

Sexual Orientation: The deep-down, inner feeling of who we are attracted or "oriented" to sexually, erotically, and emotionally. Some categories of sexual orientation include lesbian, gay (attracted to some members of the same sex), bisexual (attracted to some members of both binary genders), straight (attracted to some members of the opposite sex), and asexual (not sexually attracted to others).

Sexual Identity: This is what we call ourselves in terms of our sexuality. Such labels include "lesbian," "gay," "bisexual," "bi," "bicurious," "pansexual," "pomosexual," "queer," "questioning," "undecided," "undetermined," "heterosexual," "straight," "asexual," and others. Our sexual behavior and how we define ourselves (identity) is a choice; sexual orientation is not a choice.

Biological Sex: This can be considered our "packaging" and is determined by our chromosomes (such as XX or XY), our hormones (estrogen/progesterone or testosterone), and our internal and external genitalia (vulva, clitoris, vagina, penis, testicles).

Gender: A set of social, psychological, and emotional traits, often influenced by societal expectations that classify an individual as feminine, masculine, androgynous, or other. Gender is often linked with sex, but this is inaccurate because sex refers to birth genitalia and/or chromosomes or hormones, and gender refers to social and emotional feelings and norms.

Gender Expression: This refers to an individual's physical characteristics, behaviors, and presentation, such as appearance, dress, mannerisms, speech patterns, and social interactions that are linked, traditionally, to either masculinity or femininity. Gender expression is not an indication of sexual orientation.

Gender Identity: This is how we identify ourselves in terms of our gender. Identities may be male, female, androgynous, bi-gender, transgender, and others.

Gender Non-Conforming or Gender Variant: An identity for a person who has gender characteristics and/or behaviors that do not conform to traditional or societal binary gender expectations. Gender non-conforming people may or may not identify as lesbian, gay, bisexual, transgender, or queer.

Intersectionality: A concept often used in critical theories to describe the ways in which oppressive institutions are interconnected and cannot be examined separately from one another.

Healthcare Disparities: Differences in access to or availability of facilities and services.

Health Status Disparities: The variation in rates of disease occurrence and disabilities between socioeconomic and/or geographically-defined population groups.

Resources

Bornstein, K.. (1995). *Gender outlaw: On men, women, and the rest of us.* New York: Vintage.

Boylan, J. F. (2013). *Stuck in the middle with you: A memoir of parenting in three genders.* New York: Crown.

Bridges, K. M. (2011). *Reproducing race: An ethnography of pregnancy as a site of racialization.* Berkeley, CA: University of California Press.

Brill, S.A. (2001). *The queer parent's primer: A lesbian and gay families' guide to navigating the straight world.* Oakland, CA: New Harbinger Publications.

Nelson, A. (2011). *Body and soul: The Black Panther Party and the fight against medical discrimination.* Minneapolis, MN: University of Minnesota Press.

Pepper, R. (2005). *The ultimate guide to pregnancy for lesbians: How to stay sane and care for yourself from preconception through birth.* San Francisco: Cleis.

Supporting Families through the Adoption Process
by Laura Furniss

One vitally important and often overlooked way a family is formed is through adoption. Like any other family, there is obviously a child and at least one parent involved. However, with adoptive families, two sets of parents are involved, and both have very distinct needs and emotional experiences when adoption has been chosen. First, we have the birth parents, who are the ones who set in motion the adoption with the choice they make to place their child for adoption. The second important figures in the adoption triad are, of course, the adoptive parents.

A word of caution; if you are supporting a family through adoption, know who your client is—the birth parent or the adoptive parent. I do not recommend that you be the doula for both, as it is hard to remain neutral if things become tense and conflict arises during the course of the birth and placement of the child. I recommend that birth parents and adoptive parents have their own separate doulas, who can then focus on their needs completely and in an unbiased way.

The birth parent experiences:

- ✓ Insensitive comments and opinions about the choice they have made for their child.

- ✓ Need to bond with and say goodbye to the baby before transferring the baby to the adoptive parents.

- ✓ Sensitive birth support (respect for role as parents, respect for desires regarding the birth plan, and transfer).

✓ Understanding and acknowledgment that they ARE parents, and an adoptive placement does not take this away.

✓ Choice to spend time with/hold/nurse the baby immediately after the birth and during hospital stay.

✓ Honoring choices on when and how to transfer the baby to adoptive parents.

✓ Honoring of the right to change their mind and parent.

✓ Grief and loss.

The adoptive parent experience:

✓ Possible lack of time to prepare, if they are chosen after or close to the time of birth.

✓ Insensitive comments about the choice to adopt or personal journey that has led them there.

✓ Need to have uninterrupted time to bond with the baby after placement.

✓ Uncertainty and fear about adoption going through or birth parent changing their mind.

✓ Baby blues or postpartum depression (yes, adoptive parents can experience this, too), and lack of understanding from others.

✓ Lack of support from others at the hospital and when the baby comes home.

✓ Grief and loss, including mixed and bittersweet feelings involving joy at being parents, yet still feeling the pain of their own struggles with infertility/miscarriage/death of a baby or child.

Recommendations as you doula the birth parents:

✓ Use sensitive language of their choosing (birth-mom or first mom or dad – ask their preference, making a choice, or choosing adoption versus giving the baby up for adoption, etc.).

✓ Honor their wishes regarding when and how to meet and bond with their baby, whether it is to hold the baby right after birth, nurse or bottle-feed, pump and donate to the adoptive parents, or have the baby taken out of the room to give them some time to prepare before holding the baby. Encourage birthparents who are reluctant to hold the baby to do so. Whatever they decide, honor and respect their wishes, and advocate for them.

✓ They are parents. Age and circumstances do not matter. Respect that they are parents.

✓ Honor decision to nurse or not nurse—parent's choice!

✓ Help them make a plan for transfer to adoptive parents – when, where, and how, ritual or ceremony? Do they want to transfer before leaving the hospital? Do they want to leave the hospital with the baby and arrange a transfer ceremony elsewhere? There may be a waiting period before parents can legally sign paperwork terminating their legal rights, so know what this time period is and support the birth parents' plans and wishes.

✓ Honor their right to change their mind and choose to parent (NOT keep or not keep) their child. Help them prepare: resources, supplies, referrals, etc. Help them break the news to the potential adoptive family, if they want you to.

✓ Acknowledge and validate grief and loss over choice, even if they feel it is the best choice. Parents need to first spend time with and bond with and say hello to the baby, so they can then say goodbye. Honor their grief and how difficult this process is.

Recommendations as you doula the adoptive parents:

✓ Use sensitive language of the parents' choosing (i.e., parent/mom/ dad, birth parent versus real parent).

✓ Ask them what else they need and offer to help them fill last-minute needs. Ask if they want to nurse. Yes, adoptive parents can do this! Give them information and support as needed.

✓ Honor their space to hold and bond with the baby. Don't ask to hold the baby. The baby is grieving and needs both time to bond with birth parents, and uninterrupted time with the adoptive parents.

✓ Validate their fears about the birth parent changing their minds, allow them to feel what they feel. Help them navigate and honor the birth parent's wishes regarding bonding, breastfeeding, and transfer. If the birth parent does choose to parent rather than place the baby with the family, be with them, and acknowledge and validate their grief. Let them grieve!

✓ Acknowledge and validate confusing feelings of joy at being parents intermingled with guilt at taking someone else's baby, grief that they could not birth their child, and the difficulty of their journey to become parents.

✓ Help arrange household help/help with meals, and childcare for older children once the baby comes home. Adoptive parents cherish and need this help too, just like any parent who has given birth.

✓ Allow grief regarding infertility/miscarriage/losses that are still present or freshly reopened during this time.

Supporting Families through the Surrogacy Process
by Laura Furniss

Another way families are formed is through surrogacy. Similar to adoption, two parties are involved, with their own distinct needs and emotional experiences throughout the surrogacy experience. The surrogate is one part of this process, as the person who chooses to carry the child for the parents that have not been able to. The second important figures in the surrogacy process are, of course, the intended parents.

The surrogate experiences:

✓ Insensitive comments and opinions about the choice to be a surrogate.

✓ Pressure to be successful in achieving and sustaining pregnancy.

✓ Loneliness.

✓ Need for physical and emotional support during pregnancy and postpartum.

✓ Sensitive birth support (respect for surrogate's role and desires regarding birth plan).

✓ Choice to pump colostrum and/or breast milk for parents or to donate.

✓ Grief and loss.

The intended parent experience:

- ✓ Possibly being far away from the surrogate and unable to participate in prenatal appointments and other parts of the pregnancy.

- ✓ Insensitive comments about choice to use a surrogate or personal journey that has led them there.

- ✓ Baby blues or postpartum depression (yes, intended parents can experience this too), and lack of understanding from others.

- ✓ Lack of knowledge about pregnancy, birth, and parenting.

- ✓ Lack of support from others at the hospital and when the baby comes home.

- ✓ Grief and loss.

Recommendations as you doula the surrogate:

- ✓ Use sensitive language of their choosing (surrogate versus surrogate mother; ask their preference, surrogate or surro baby versus their baby, giving the parents' the baby back versus giving up their baby).

- ✓ Offer to go with the surrogate to appointments so they do not have to go alone. Many times, the intended parents are not close enough to be there.

- ✓ Focus on the surrogate during the birth and postpartum, as the intended parents are often the focus of attention. Suggest a birth photographer, as this can help with the healing process postpartum. They can go back and see what everyone was doing during the birth. Offer to sit down with them afterward and write their birth story with them.

- ✓ Offer to set up a meal train or other help for when the surrogate goes home. Encourage visits from friends. Surrogates are often forgotten because there is no baby to focus on. They need attention and help, as well.

✓ Surrogates are often seen as selfless for choosing to be a surrogate and face people who believe they chose this, so they need to deal with it, but they still have very real physical and emotional needs. They appreciate and desire offers for help, comfort, self-care, and other needs.

✓ Encourage midwives and obstetricians to follow up with the surrogate. Again, surrogates' needs are often overlooked when there is no baby to care for.

✓ Assess for signs of perinatal and postpartum depression or other mood disorders. Talk to them about this, so they know it can and does sometimes happen.

✓ Honor choice to pump for the baby, or to donate. Refer to a lactation consultant as appropriate.

✓ Acknowledge and validate grief and loss. Surrogates can grieve over the loss of the baby they carried, even though they knew they would say goodbye. Also, surrogates grieve when they are not chosen as the surrogate for subsequent pregnancies, for any reason.

Recommendations as you doula the intended parents:

✓ Use sensitive language of their choosing (intended parents, other).

✓ Ask them what else they need and offer to help them fill last-minute needs. Ask if they want to nurse. Yes, this is possible! Give them information and support as needed.

✓ Honor their space to hold and bond with the baby. Don't ask to hold the baby. The baby is grieving (remember, the baby has been inside of and bonded with the voice, smells, etc. of someone else) and needs time to bond with the parents. A helpful hint: The surrogate and intended parents can use belly buds during the pregnancy to help the baby hear their voices.

✓ Suggest pregnancy and birthing classes and parenting classes, as well as counseling to help them process through fears and grief related to losses.

✓ Assess for mood disorders and offer information about this.

✓ Acknowledge and validate confusing feelings of joy at being parents intermingled with grief that they could not birth their child, and the difficulty of their journey to become parents.

✓ Help arrange household help, help with meals, and childcare for older children once the baby comes home. Intended parents cherish and need this help too, just like any parent who has given birth.

✓ Allow grief regarding infertility/miscarriage/losses that are still present or freshly reopened during this time.

Written in collaboration with Amber Campanelli from Montana Surrogacy (www.montanasurro.com)

The Transition to Dadhood

by Dr. Jay Warren

Nowadays, dads play an essential role in prenatal care, birth preparation, and in labor and delivery. New fathers are also now expected to be active caregivers in the first days, weeks, and months of their child's life—bathing, bottle-feeding, diaper changing, clothing, soothing, cuddling, putting down to sleep, playing—all the things parents do to care for a newborn, as they should. But this wasn't always the case.

Today, it is common for us to see images of men massaging lower backs in labor and catching babies in birth tubs. But not too long ago, the images we saw were of men passing out cigars in the hospital waiting room after hearing from the doctor that "It's a boy!" or "It's a girl!" Generations ago, men were not a part of pregnancy, birth, or early parenting. The father was relegated to the role of the *provider/protector* of the family unit, and when the child was older, the role of the *disciplinarian* was added and then maybe the role of the *teacher/mentor*.

So much has changed for the better.

My own father was part of a pilot program in the early 1970s, where they experimented with "allowing" fathers to be in the delivery room. My birth fell within a 3-month trial period at St. John's Hospital in Los Angeles, CA. But my father almost wasn't there. On the night of my birth, my mom's regular OB wasn't available, and the OB on call was not supportive of this new program. As the family story goes, my dad and this OB were yelling at each other in the hallway about whether or not he would be permitted into the delivery room when my mom shouted at them, "Would you two figure this out later? I'm going to have a baby!" My dad was allowed in, and I was born with him there beside my mom.

Fast forward to me becoming a dad: I went to every prenatal visit (except for one, when I was too sick to go), and I was actively involved in the birth planning and decision-making.

I was present at my son's birth, who was born at home. It was just me, Mama, the midwife, and the doula. I got to catch him. I got to cut the cord. I got to be the first one he "meconium pooed" on.

Only a few weeks into parenting life, I spent my first day caring for my son alone. Was I nervous? You bet! We did great together, and I texted plenty of "proof of life" pictures throughout that day to keep Mama calm at work. I remember feeling so relieved when Mama got home that night, though, to relieve me from baby duty. And while I enjoyed sitting back and watching her doting on our son, I also enjoyed basking in the glow of a dad's job well done.

As our parenting lifestyle unfolded, with her work schedule and mine as it was, I spent half the week with my newborn son. Full days together, just us two. And it didn't feel unusual or abnormally stressful to me doing this because I was "just the dad." It just was. I enjoyed doing it and felt grateful that I got to do it.

But I hear so many stories in my practice that the level of a dad's involvement with the baby in the first few months is very different. Many fathers-to-be we see in our prenatal wellness center are going to the birth education classes, attending prenatal visits, and are there at the birth. But I hear from the new moms afterward that their spouses are not engaged in newborn care, despite their efforts to get the dad involved. I hear comments like, "He won't help with anything since he says I'm the one breastfeeding and knows how to do everything" or even, "My husband? Oh, he's useless. He has no idea what to do." The new dads are described to me as detached, uninvolved, uninterested, oblivious, incapable, inconvenienced, frustrated, and annoyed.

Now in some cases, I'm sure that's true. But the majority of the new dads I've worked with do not feel this way. Are they frustrated? Yes. But not detached or uninterested. Annoyed? Maybe. But not for the reasons their spouses think.

The frustration we feel comes from the pressure of the unclear expectations placed upon us as new dads and not really knowing how to fulfill them. We don't have any generational experience to draw upon because our grandfathers, great-grandfathers, and beyond were not involved. And we have little cultural reference because this current version of what an active father actually looks and feels like is so new. So, we are lacking the resources and support we need to help us navigate this major life transition into Dadhood. And as frustrating as that is, what is worse is that we feel like we are letting our families down.

But that too can change for the better.

The first thing that we can do to help new dads is to make sure an open dialog between Mom and Dad about what new parenthood will look like and the expectations that each brings to it is happening. I've found that the birth education classes we teach start a similar type of dialog for couples. However, it usually only focuses on the last trimester of pregnancy and the onset of labor, but then it stops at birth.

If moms and dads continued this exploration of what new parenthood is going to look like for them once the baby has arrived and about the expectations each one has for the first days, weeks, and months together, then so much strife could be avoided. Parents-to-be should have discussions about: How are the tasks of nighttime diaper changes, laundry, meal prep, and dishes going to be divided or who is responsible for each? Who is going to which appointments with the baby? Who's going to manage the grandparents? Who's making sure the bills are paid on time? Who's going back to work and when? And then what's supposed to happen when the other walks through the door from work at the end of the day? What does that (and so much more with early parenting) all look like?

Getting both Mom and Dad on the same page is essential for their family unit to be strong and functional during this significant transition from couplehood into parenthood. A united Mom and Dad care for their baby so much better together.

But I feel that new dads also need support from other men as well through this transition to Dadhood. A kind of support that can only come from other men. In my experience, men in a group class setting with their spouses sitting next to them share only a superficial layer of what's really going on inside them. For generations, men have been taught that when it comes to their family, they need to provide, protect, and lead. I don't feel that any of these roles are bad ones to assume, and I believe that being strong within each one of them will indeed serve our families. But what it means to be a *protector, provider,* and *leader* in today's family is much different than what it meant to generations of fathers long ago. The roles that were passed on to us by past generations need a modern upgrade. I don't pretend that I know just how those roles should be upgraded exactly. But I feel new dads need ways to explore this and figure it out together.

By being part of a few men's groups myself, I've seen how the group sharing dynamic shifts when it is "men only." If a safe space is set up, if ground rules are established and boundaries are consistently maintained, then I've seen men open up in powerful ways that do not happen in mixed groups. Men share their frustration about not relating well with their kids and their sadness about the level of disconnect they feel with their wives. They admit their despair in feeling that they are losing their marriage and screwing up their children despite trying everything they can to keep it all together. Sometimes this is the first time that a man has not only said these things out loud, but the first time they have admitted to and been honest with themselves about these feelings.

Our new dads need this kind of space to be able to open up and show our chinks in our armor without worrying that our family will think less of us. When trust is built, vulnerability can be shared. When safety is felt, worries and fears can be shared. Statements of "I never seem to be able to calm the baby down quickly enough so then she swoops in frustrated with me that she has to do it again" is met with some new tips and tools that might do the trick next time. Confessions of "I just don't feel that connected to my baby yet, not like her mom does [...] and I'm worried I'm not going to love them enough" is answered by "I went through the same thing. It's normal. Don't worry, it'll kick in soon enough."

When you're overwhelmed, and so inside your own bubble, a simple reassurance that what you're going through is normal, and that we've all been there too, can make a huge difference.

Ironically, isn't it when we finally admit these fears, being open and vulnerable about what is challenging us, that it usually brings our family closer together? But most men have never been taught how to share deep feelings openly, and we are afraid that we will disappoint our closest loved ones. So, when the overwhelm of new parenthood hits us, we try to compartmentalize it and control it ourselves. If that doesn't work, we isolate ourselves, so no one sees our failure. But when we pretend the problem doesn't exist, it doesn't stop us from feeling the pain of it. We dig ourselves into a deeper and deeper hole with many unhealthy consequences, for ourselves and our family. But we're not alone.

So, in a "New Dads Group," having a safe place to talk about whatever is on your chest that night has the potential to create powerful changes in not only that man's life but in his family as well. Of course, a "men's only" group is not the only place this can happen. I've just seen that sometimes it is easier for men to start opening up with a group of relative strangers, but with whom they share a common bond: Dadhood. Then, with practice and repetition, the hope is this new ability to express vulnerability and honesty is brought back home and shared within the family as well. Even if the monthly meeting is a place to "blow off steam" and not feel so alone, it will help the family be just a little bit healthier.

The transition into Dadhood can be an overwhelming experience for men, just as the transition into motherhood can be for women. But we don't have to feel so alone in figuring it out. Communicating and managing expectations is the key to both Mom and Dad feeling supported, cared for, and loved as they navigate their way in becoming a happy, happy family together.

Possibilities: When Life Includes a Family Member with a Disability

by Jamie Lee Marks

Handicapped, disabled, impaired, crippled, lame, retarded, idiot, imbecile, moron, special needs, exceptional, diverse, midget, little person, low incidence, high-functioning, trainable, teachable, tolerable, dumb, vegetable, gifted, differently-abled, spastic, pervasive developmental disorder, mentally impaired, emotionally disturbed, deaf, mute, blind, sightless…

Life as a Professional

For 30 plus years, I have worked in a field where titles and acronyms dance on a calendar of perception, switching positions and substituting word and letter partners to outlive its predecessor, at least long enough to be part of some lasting text or acceptable identity. In my teenage years, I volunteered at camps and events for children and adults with disabilities. It is a natural inclination to categorize people according to abilities, much like the events they competed in. It was interesting to me that even within the broad groupings, there were unspoken splits within, depending on origin, type, and functioning level. The athletes I worked within the early Para-Olympic games hung in self-chosen groups based on acquired (amputee, spinal cord injury, etc.) or congenital (cerebral palsy, spina bifida) labels.

People found it easier to use vague generalizations rather than complicated medical terms to describe themselves or their children: on the spectrum, physically involved, tactually defensive. Umbrella terms may be further divided by different values, traditions, and communications. There are individuals who are part of deaf culture, and individuals who are part of the blind community. Where do those with dual-sensory loss, or "deaf/blind," fit in? Are they all part of the "Sensory" category? In the early 90s, when I was an O.I./O.H.I teacher (that stands for *Orthopedic Impairment/Other Health Impaired),* students who did not "fit" into other categories were placed in my self-contained classroom. This included children with autism, who were medically fragile, had immunity issues, and hybrid conditions that could not be clearly identified. This was also an era of implementing early intervention programs, inclusion, and home-based family development programs.

When I say that labels and acronyms dance at dizzying speeds, I am not kidding. As a young, married without children, special education teacher, I would lead my IEP meetings with parents of young children who got OT, PT, SLP, AdPE, GE, SSP, VI, HI (Occupational Therapy, Physical Therapy, Speech-Language Pathology, Adapted Physical Education, General Education, Student Support Personnel, Vision Impairments, Hearing Impairments). And just to make sure we re-used letters as much as possible for continued confusion, students who received early intervention services were part of the E.I.P, and they could not have an I.E.P. (Individualized Education Program). It all made perfect sense to me, and I explained it perfectly at the meetings and conferences with the parents. And then, I had a baby.

Real Life

My mother was legally blind by the time she was 11. She was the first in the family to have an actual diagnosis: retinitis pigmentosa. For our family, this diagnosis included the loss of night/low light vision, loss of peripheral vision (like tunnel vision), decreased depth perception, sensitivity to glare, and longer adjustment to lighting changes. In our family, it is also characterized by an increased sense of humor, padded legs, and particularly hard heads. We have traced this genetic tradition back six generations. While not formally diagnosed, we had relatives and family members that were "messy housekeepers," "afraid to go out at night," and "clumsy." This was not the case with my mother. We grew up in Brooklyn, and it wasn't until we moved to Long Island when I was 10 that I noticed that my mother did not drive. We traveled by bus, train, foot, and bicycle. She never complained about not being able to drive, or her vision changes over time, or even how my Japanese/Korean father would introduce her as "My wife, she's blind." She taught me to be an ambassador for change and to not get stuck in verbiage. To this day, when someone asks me what my guide dog is for, I pick a term. On Mondays, I say, "I am legally blind." On Tuesdays, I may state, "I have a vision impairment." If it is raining, I use "Low Vision." Twice a month, I enthusiastically proclaim to inquiring minds, "I am Partially Sighted." I have a friend who tells people that he is "visually inconvenienced"; I'll have to mix that one in somehow.

For many years, I was very good at blending in my sighted world. I drove for twenty-some years, taught, shopped, had a family, and a house. My first pregnancy was complicated because I had been given the wrong medicine in my prenatal vitamin refill. It was mistakenly filled with *Motrin* instead of *Materna Pre*. I took 800 mg a day of Motrin for about 3 weeks in my first trimester before I noticed the tiny word on the pill one evening. This may or may not have been the first time I had ever thought that my vision had changed. Truly, it was small print, and I didn't have my glasses on most times I took my vitamin. However, for the rest of my pregnancy, I saw a prenatal specialist. I worried about all the things that could go wrong. The parents of my students had shared their stories with me on occasion, and I had visions of tiny babies hooked up to machines, non-verbal toddlers pulling themselves around on their elbows, me pouring formula into a funnel connected by a tube into a button surgically attached to the baby's stomach.

I had a wonderful midwife for the birth, and a best-friend doula, just a phone call away. I had my family and felt very supported. I did not acknowledge my vision changes, nor did I consider my daughter's vision at this time, although I felt well-prepared for just about anything, (being a teacher trained in early intervention, I had lots of experience with babies and young children). Oh, it is a whole new ballgame with your own. Breastfeeding was difficult, and I could feel the pressure of not succeeding and disappointing my parents, especially my father (that's for a different day). That awesome routine and perfectly structured day of enrichment, love, and laughter disguised itself as tears, meltdowns, and fear.

Most of what I felt was typical new-mom stuff. Over time, things settled down. I had a lactation consultant, a very good pump, and all went forward. I was back at work six-weeks later, pumping twice a day in a little janitor's closet near my classroom, taking naps at red-lights, and looking forward to summer break. My baby became used to nightlights and my little flashlight that I would use to check on her in the dark. I subconsciously created contrast and made sure surfaces were cleared and clean, visually and tactually. Other than that, my vision was not "inconveniencing" me.

By the time I was pregnant with my son, four years later, things were different. The pregnancy was again complicated due to me having "Fifth's Disease" in my first trimester. Once again, I was in the care of a prenatal specialist most of my second and third trimester. The risk to the baby meant weekly visits and ultrasounds that could focus on each chamber of his heart. If it looked enlarged or at risk to burst, immediate termination would be necessary, regardless of the age/stage of the baby. Each week, I left early from school and drove to the doctor, wondering if I would have a baby inside me tomorrow. Meanwhile, my daughter was struggling with emotions and fine motor tasks at preschool. She cried more than usual and slept with the lights on. My vision was changing, and I was beginning to make subtle adaptations. I didn't drive at night as much; I was very organized and kept travel areas clear of toys. I asked my mother about vision when she was my age and how it interfered or complicated motherhood. I worried about having a wild boy who would run off and hide in department store racks, leave matchbox cars and Lego traps, and easily slip out into the night in the teenage years because he knew Mom wouldn't be able to see or catch him. I begged for those dilemmas every week, laying on the exam table with the yucky stuff on my belly, staring at the monitor and listening to the percussion of life.

Shortly after my son was born, my daughter was diagnosed with retinitis pigmentosa. At the time, we knew there would be a chance, but we did not know until many years later that the probability was 50%. She was five. My husband and my father had noticed that she had difficulty seeing in the dark when she was about 3 or 4. She had some fine-motor issues and struggled with schoolwork at preschool. We wondered if it was the Motrin. We wondered if it was her highly emotional, overly sensitive, transition-resistant behavior. Could it be the new-baby adjustment thing? Perhaps she can see in the dark but just prefers the lights on. After all, Mom uses a flashlight, nightlight, and opens the blinds first thing in the morning. The answer is D: All of the above.

With the number of women affected with RP in our family, it was not a total shocker. Given that I was still driving and seeing well during the day, I had the hope that her case would not be as severe as my mom's. I had cataract surgery that year. One of the byproducts of Retinitis Pigmentosa can be early onset cataracts. I remember saying to my surgeon, "I need to nurse my son before I go in for the cataract surgery [...] Hey, I bet you don't hear that every day from your patients."

When my son was 8, and my daughter was 13, we were living in the Philadelphia area. We began doing research studies with Children's Hospital and the University of Pennsylvania for treatments for retinal diseases like retinitis pigmentosa. It was here that my son was diagnosed with RP. I was so shocked. He had no symptoms. He was a boy; I already had one child with it. What kind of odds were these? My brother, my cousins, everyone in my generation who had kids—not one single case. I have two. At this time, I was no longer driving; I stopped teaching, I had begun my Vision Rehabilitation Therapy: learning Braille, learning to travel with a white cane, and using public transportation.

I was feeling VERY visually inconvenienced. I was very depressed, and I stayed in bed for two days. I thought about all the preachy sentiments I had said to the parents of my students, all the copies of "Welcome to Holland" that I handed out at faculty meetings and parent nights. I thought about all the loss, and sacrifice, and compromise, and control-giving I had experienced over these ten years, the strain on my marriage, my resentment toward my wonderful mom, because I could not be as accepting and embracing of this situation as she was, and now, I have sentenced my children to the same dark cell.

I would love to say that my mom flung open my bedroom door and unapologetically dragged me to my feet and convinced me with one golden phrase; "It's not a death sentence," I suddenly had an epiphany, and then everything was okay. I would like to say that I instantly found the strength and inner voice to be the best role model, pillar of independence, leader of confident living, and creative, long-term planner. The truth is, it has been a long process of grieving, smiling, tripping forward, and leaning on others.

So, what have I learned and what do I yearn to share?

✓ **The label**

> Don't get hung up on it either way. Having a diagnosis is a starting point and gives some framework. It is not a solid definition, but it has some identity merit.

✓ **Family**

> They bring you strength, and in the next breath, bring you to your knees. The comfort that comes from knowing where you came from can be a nice outline for your own book, or it can just be irony. If those related by blood can't be relied on, find another.

✓ **Access the resources**

> There are people who specialize in EVERYTHING and ONE THING: working with families, babies, siblings, teachers, therapists, and so on for every scenario, even if it means piecing different subject matter experts together to form a beautiful quilt of collaboration. These teams become the well-constructed family for today and tomorrow.

✓ **Grieve**

Any outcome that is less than the perceived expectation can be considered. Regardless of how unrealistic it may be, the notion, the physical reality, and all the connections in between will need to be re-adjusted. Grieve the loss and fill in the spaces.

✓ **Love and protection are not the same things**

The most handicapping condition of all is overprotection. Easier said than done. But, from day one, consider the benefits of exploring options for learning, choice-making, creative communications, and building trust.

✓ **Expand the senses**

A multi-sensory approach paves the path. The sentiment, "it's the journey, not the destination" may have some very scenic routes. There are 7 senses; you know the first five (hearing, seeing, tasting, touching, smelling). Those may be compromised; that is when the other two come to the rescue: sense of HUMOR and sense of ADVENTURE.

✓ **Realize the POSSIBILITIES**

The author of this book once told me the story of her young son and his reaction to seeing a man with a disability. He asked her, "Does that man have a possibility?"

"Yes," she replied, "He does."

I love this word for all its meanings and all its potential. I use this word in lieu of other terms when I am writing or presenting. I say, "I work with people who have possibilities." I teach students with multiple possibilities. It is the most liberating label I know.

Loss and Grief

by Ann Grauer

Of all the topics that doulas need to know about, grief and loss are the ones that cause the most concern. We work with beginnings: new baby, new family, new roles. We expect to know about the "starts" in life. It is a cruel irony that all beginnings also involve endings.

The Hallmark Card version of having a baby is that they live happily ever after. As we know, this is not how real, messy life works. When a baby enters the family, the types of grief and loss experienced often include:

- ✓ Loss of freedom

- ✓ Loss of former sense of self

- ✓ Grief over the money situation

- ✓ Loss of intimacy

- ✓ Loss of control

When I first started as a doula, I felt prepared to help a client with those concerns, and I hoped and prayed that I would never encounter a family with a loss of a baby. I was terrified that I wouldn't know what to say or how to act. Instead, in my first year of doula work, my own second daughter was stillborn, and I almost left the work altogether. After a time, I felt doula work call my name, and I returned with trepidation and determination. I have been blessed to work with many clients since then. Some have lost a baby; most have not. What my husband and I wanted during our loss is not what every parent needs or desires—there is no magical answer for how to work with families experiencing grief, but there are definitely things that can help.

We expect that when change occurs, there will be an adjustment time. Our clients are already experiencing huge change. When grief and loss are added into the mix, they have gone from an expected type of change to one they never wanted: losing their baby. Never underestimate how deeply this can affect parents and their family and friends.

Working with new families requires doulas to be honest with themselves. In regard to grief, here is something to think about; how comfortable are you in regards to death and dying? If you have avoided these topics, or are feeling anxious about them, you will need to do a little work in order to serve families who encounter loss. Learning to become more familiar with your own response to these important topics will allow you to be present with a family instead of preoccupied with your own fears at that time. Frankly, your personal development in this area will serve you throughout your lifetime, as well as your career.

So, if your client experiences a loss, what is your role? Like most anything else in doula work, it depends on what the client wants. Some will cut off the relationship with the doula and not wish to see them again. This is known as transference and can happen when someone goes through a large, sudden change. It doesn't mean the family blames the doula for what happened, but rather, they are a symbol of what has been lost, and they cannot handle it. Seeing us is too painful. For the doula, this can feel devastating. However, their reaction is not about you.

Other families will hold tightly to the doula, and seek their help and presence. In this instance, the doula follows the client's lead, while also remembering the bigger picture. Our clients still have the same basic needs they had before: there may be physical changes that the mother is experiencing, such as lochia, dealing with breastmilk, etc. They still need to eat and to sleep or rest.

The best approach is usually to go to the client and say, "I am here for you." Then, be still and present. Let yourself get comfortable during long silences with a client who is crying. Or, you may need to settle in with a client who is, almost robotically, listing off things that must be done. No two people respond to loss in the same way. If you come to them with the approach that nothing they can say or do can cause you to not want to walk alongside them, that is enough.

Your organizational and practical skills are often put to work. You may find that you are spending time helping the family to organize thoughts or creating lists that need to be ticked. The client's family may be making decisions that are overwhelming and confusing. You can be the notetaker and write things down so that they will be able to read what happened and who said what. Often, friends and family will bring food, and the client will be grateful later when you are able to provide them with information on who brought what and when. You are bearing witness and providing context as they move through this foggy time.

As with any doula work, we go back to the basics. Your job will be providing support that is Practical, Informational, and Emotional (PIE). The client will let you know what they need from you and when. Using PIE as a foundation, here are a few ideas.

Practical

✓ Organizating and/or preparing meals.

✓ Taking notes as needed.

✓ Being present.

✓ Assisting parents and/or other professionals with creating tangible memories (these can include printing and framing pictures, handprints, etc.).

✓ Helping the client to care for themselves.

✓ Attending any memorial service or funeral.

✓ Assisting with contacting others who need to know (including email lists, etc.).

Informational

✓ Sharing information on grief and loss for family (info for all members, if possible).

✓ Having contact information for resources that may be of help at this time: counselors/therapists, support groups, websites, and even perhaps names of other parents who are willing to be contacted.

✓ Helping parents sort through their options, including how to share their wishes with their loved ones (i.e., do they wish to pack baby items themselves versus others doing it for them).

Emotional

✓ Listening.

✓ Affirming and normalizing the client's feelings.

✓ Bearing witness to this time.

✓ Offering a hug or just a hand on their back.

✓ Reminding them that they are not alone.

✓ Listening actively or reflectively as they speak.

✓ Helping them find their voice.

Afterward

Dates are all important to clients, and remembering them can be so helpful. The baby's due date, birthday, date of death—all can are meaningful, and when they come around, many people do not remember them. Set a reminder to send the client a message or card around those times. Just saying "thinking of you" is enough.

While you are at it, remind yourself to check in on the client monthly, then at three to six-month intervals in that first year afterward. You never know how much your reaching out can mean to them.

Taking Care of You

You are doing essential work, and it will be important for you to have someone to speak with. Another doula can be a great sounding board, and they will have an understanding of your feelings from their own experience. Sometimes, we need someone who can listen to us professionally and help us process our thoughts and feelings. This is when knowing an excellent counselor or therapist can be helpful. None of us are unphased when working with families who have lost a baby.

Some doulas find that writing or painting helps them to work through their own feelings. Many seek ways to honor the families who have lost babies. One doula found that planting bulbs in her garden for each baby was soothing. They are the first flowers to bloom in the spring and remind her of the circle of life.

As you begin to think about working with a family experiencing loss, you may be concerned that you are not ready. That's okay; no one is ever truly prepared. Remember to go back to being present ("I'm here for you") and then to listen.

The Perinatal Period and Sexuality

by Natashia Fuksman

✓ "I can't look down there yet. It's way too much!"

✓ "At the end of the day, my partner wants to touch me. I have nothing left—I am all touched out!"

✓ "I feel triumphant after giving birth, and very sexual. But I'm embarrassed to say, my partner has lost *his* sex drive."

✓ "My breasts right now are for my baby. I don't even care about looking at them or want my partner to look at them in any other way."

✓ "I gave explicit instructions to my partner to position himself at my head. I was way too worried that he wouldn't enjoy me the same if he saw our baby coming out."

We tend to not talk about the sexual experience of the perinatal period (pregnancy, birth, and postpartum) in our culture. In fact, there is a "splitting" mentality when it comes to these two parts of the self, that is between the sexual self and the parenting self. It is as if after birth, one's sexuality becomes nonexistent. There is a common myth that the baby will "kill your sex life." Outside of this myth, there really isn't much that is spoken of in our culture about the relationship between the perinatal time and one's sexuality. Unfortunately, this "splitting" invites a lack of information, leaving new parents in the dark, setting them up for experiences that may be surprising, confusing, and/or shocking.

In fact, there is a strong and complex relationship between sexuality and the perinatal period. As a sex therapist who specializes in working with individuals and couples who are actively parenting young children, I can attest that there are indeed a large range of experiences both biological mothers and partners have regarding arousal, sexual identity, fantasy, stimulation, and the ever-evolving experience of intimacy. The good news is that you don't have to know it all! And yet, you may be curious.

From a biological perspective, it's significant to note that all of a woman's sexual organs are part of her reproductive system. These organs are creating, building, and functioning towards the life and birth of her baby. From the moment of conception, her sexual/reproductive system is functioning in both new and older, familiar ways. Logically, this impacts her identity, including her sexual self. With the very same organs that comprise her reproductive system, the mother is able to produce life while simultaneously experiencing pleasure through desire, arousal, and contact.

Part of what may cause the "splitting" is that it is complex to acknowledge and understand one organ having more than one main function. This difficulty in comprehending the multiple functions of an organ is demonstrated in the language we use to describe function and pleasure in a woman's reproductive system. We use different terms to refer to where a woman experiences penetration and where she gives birth, even though they are one and the same place. When speaking of penetration, this body part is commonly referred to as a "vaginal canal." This is because it is a canal portion of her vagina. The vaginal canal has an opening at the base of her vagina. There is a tubular shape that has soft mushy tissue, creating folds and can get wonderfully moist and engorged when she is aroused or stimulated in this area.

The other end of this canal ends at her cervix or the "neck" (Latin root) of her uterus. The cervix has a very small opening leading further inside her body, to the rest of her uterus, where the baby is gestating in a well-protected, sterile environment. The uterus is well protected from anything penetrating beyond the vaginal canal through the smallness of the opening in the cervix and a layer of mucus that forms all around the cervix, barring bacteria from passing this "wall" of mucus. So, the vaginal canal is really this incredible place where so much happens.

It's interesting to note the vaginal canal is often renamed when the mother is giving birth. Upon giving birth, the more common term for this part of a woman's body is the "birth canal," as if there may be another canal in her vagina that has the purpose of birthing. Here, in the language, we see the splitting. Calling this canal two separate terms—one associated with penetration (and hopefully, pleasure) and one with birth—gives the illusion, if not misconception, that we are actually talking about two separate parts of a woman's body. The reality, however, is this is the same place in a woman's body. The place that actually has many abilities. The vagina is a place where one can experience pleasure, penetration, conception, and giving birth. What a powerful organ!

When realizing that we are speaking of the same body parts, it may make even more sense to note that during the perinatal period, some of the sensations and/or experiences with the newborn may be sensationally familiar to the mother because they are happening in the same parts of the woman's body. The sensations may have a correlation with feelings that are connected to the mother's first or most prominent experiences around these body parts (i.e., the vagina, breasts, etc.). This may be experienced in both conscious and unconscious ways. If it is conscious, it can happen in the form of flashbacks associated with this area of her body, or associated with something about the process of pregnancy, birth, breastfeeding, etc. When unconscious, feelings or reactions arise without the mother understanding why she is experiencing *these* feelings when amidst her newborn.

For example, a client of mine, whom we will call Veronica, was struggling with breastfeeding because of sexual abuse centered around her breasts she had experienced as a teenager. That abuse occurred 20 years before Veronica had her firstborn, and even so, each time she breastfed her newborn, she struggled with flashbacks of her earlier trauma. This was confusing and retraumatizing for Veronica. She had not realized during her pregnancy that her previous sexual abuse history might be triggered. She, like so many others, had split her experiences related to her sexual identity from her expectations around motherhood and her "mother body." In therapy, Veronica's work centered around understanding that her body doesn't compartmentalize her sexual self from her mother self. A big realization came one day when Veronica exclaimed, "my body is one!" and she went on to share that she now realizes how her breasts have a whole history, not just one of being a mother or being the survivor of sexual abuse. This was a big turning point for her because she was able to see that her history wouldn't be erased. Rather, she could now focus on learning skills to feel compassion for herself and care for herself whenever she would get triggered by the abuse history.

When a mother who comes into pregnancy understanding that her personal history and general sexual being will be a part of the process of her perinatal journey, we can eliminate some of the confusion and maybe even some shock, as we normalize the awareness of this time period being one of sexual development. We can care for her ever-evolving whole self and help inform some of what may be at play in her integration of her past self with her growing, present self. In Veronica's case, her doula was a key part of helping the bonding process between mother and baby. Michelle, her doula, noticed some hardship with breastfeeding. Through the trust Michelle and Veronica developed over their first couple of weeks of working together, Veronica disclosed feelings of great discomfort while breastfeeding, saying that it might be related to some "difficult" things from her history. Michelle *normalized* this. She let Veronica know that this can absolutely happen because *our bodies have memories.* She let Veronica know that she didn't need to keep suffering, that there were many options.

Michelle suggested speaking with a trained therapist to help her process what was going on and to make a plan that would help her feel better and suffer less. In this case, Michelle didn't need to know the details, yet she was a vital conduit to Veronica receiving the support she needed to create more space between her earlier trauma and what was happening for her with her baby in the present. This is just one example of a way in which the body remembers, and the brain may need some support in parsing out past from present.

There are other ways in which our brains may relate the perinatal period to our sexual selves. Relationally speaking, our own parents (or guardians) were our first models for adulthood and parenthood in particular. These models are foundational imprints deep in our psyches. We don't have to live the same way our parents did, but we have those imprints as a basis to work from. As we become parents, some portion of our conscious and/or unconscious self calls upon these early imprints. Thus, as new parents are inundated with newness, they may feel into what it was like for their parents when they were becoming parents. What do they know about how their parents felt about their bodies? How they felt about their partners? Their role as parents? Their relationship with their own sexuality? New parents will often be impacted by their own experiences of what their parents' journey through this stage of development was like. This is part of the family lifecycle, where we can see how we impact one another generationally. Again, this doesn't mean we will relive what our parents' experience was. It means we are influenced by it.

My former client, André, shared how his parents were greatly disconnected sexually when he was a young child. Prior to becoming a father, André knew sexual connection with his long-term spouse was very important because he didn't want to repeat what he knew of his parents' disconnect. Upon becoming a father, his fear of loss of connection heightened, and as a result, he began placing extra importance on connecting with his spouse. The story he knew of his parents was that after having children, his father concentrated so much on making a living for the expanded family that he became more stressed and more distant. He didn't want to become the distant, overworked father. This was something that he knew was important for him to check in about with his partner and help increase their sense of connection at this time.

When parents have deeper insight into the ways in which their family history can inform their current reality, they may make some conscious choices around how to deepen and validate connection, as opposed to automatically reenacting what happened during a previous generation. Of course, family dynamics are not always so simple or straightforward to understand. The most important point here is that as parents are becoming parents, they are both having their new and unique experiences, *and* are being influenced by their primary associations with this time period, based on their experiences in their family of origin. Just having this understanding can make an inherently overwhelming time less confusing.

There is another *relational* way in which our sexuality is impacted during the perinatal period. If the biological mother has an intimate partner, this partner will, of course, experience vicariously some of the changes she is going through. In turn, the partner will likely experience their own changes, and this will impact the biological mother. As one expands in their sexual identity, and identity overall, surely, their intimate partner will experience their own expanding and contracting in tandem.

The mother who is a solo parent will experience her own sexual-identity development. Her evolving sexual self may be informed by all of the above, as well as (but not limited to) her story of becoming a solo parent. Some things to be considered are whether she became a solo parent by choice or via loss of a partner, what the conception process was like for her, and the kind of inherent acknowledgment her support community gives to her intimate life.

A new mother may experience positive, negative, neutral, or numb feelings about her sexual self. Most commonly, a complex concoction of feelings comes up in different contexts related to sexual identity during the postpartum time period. Earlier sexual experiences may arise in the form of flashbacks; the mother may have unresolved feelings about pregnancy and/ or labor experience; she may have flashbacks of how she was treated and touched by care providers or during the birthing of her baby; she may be dealing with issues related to feeding her newborn, and this often will inform her present-day relationship with her breasts, her body overall, and her sexual identity.

How we engage with our sexual selves evolves over the lifespan. It is not stagnant. When our bodies change, we change with them. So, we can expect that mothers (and partners) postpartum will have an evolving sexual experience. Just as at any stage of development (i.e., puberty, first love, the newlywed time period, postpartum, menopause/midlife, etc.), it is extremely helpful to have safe people who can help us hold the complexity of this big time of change in our lives. Part of holding that complexity is not trying to solve it or pretend it is not there. Rather, it is to acknowledge it, accept it, and perhaps show interest or curiosity over the mother's unique experience. Part of the holding is to invite this big time of change to have a newness that is messy and confusing and filled with big love *and* grief over what was lost, all at the same time.

Here are some ideas of things to keep in mind when working with a mother postpartum:

✓ **Ask open-ended questions.**

Open-ended questions provide space for the mother to open up to you, in whatever way she desires. Things like, "Would you like to share a little about how it's been to be in your body recently?" or, "Have you noticed any points of connection with your partner lately—big or small?" She may have many things she wants to share in reference to you asking an open question. She also may have very little to say. Either way, you are planting a seed in asking. You are inviting the new mother to be curious about her experience, and this is a gift. When we are going through a new stage of development, it can and often does feel so daunting. In the newborn time period, parents can often feel anxious about all the newness and responsibility in their role as "parent," sometimes losing sight of curiosity about their whole experience. Asking an open-ended question sends a message to the mother that you acknowledge a large variety of experiences can be had and that you are interested to know about her in a unique present-day journey. It personalizes and gives room for the new mother to experience a bit of her own space—something often lacking during this time period when everyone and everything can easily be focused on giving the baby what they need.

✓ **Subtly share positive regard for what the mother is doing with her body, her energy, and her efforts to intimately bond with herself, her baby, and her family.**

> Genuine noticing statements like, "I am impressed with how you are giving yourself time to shower and just be with your body" or, "It's really neat that you and your partner take advantage of little moments to joke and connect with one another." Noticing what is happening that helps support the mother in being with her own experience and/or bond with herself, her baby, or her partner validate things that are positive and already happening. When a person is sleep-deprived and/or overwhelmed, perspective and other people's witnessing can mean so much. Genuine, positive noticing statements sprinkled here and there send messages to the mom about her new reality that is unfolding in front of everyone's eyes. These statements are validating—again, whether or not they become a source of expanded discussion.

✓ **Provide a resource list of books, blogs, sex therapists, and pelvic floor physical therapists in your area who specialize in working with women during the perinatal time period.**

> If you don't know of any sex or physical therapists who have specific knowledge about the postpartum period, you can call a perinatal therapist and ask them for referrals. The mere act of providing a resource list with information about sexuality postpartum helps parents shift from the cultural norm of splitting birth from sexuality, into accepting that sexuality, just like every other aspect of life, evolves when during life transitions, like growing one's family happens. A resource list that details care mentioning sex or sexuality also gives the mother a signal that you are someone she can speak to about issues related to her sexuality should she desire reaching out. That's huge! As a starting point for your own reference list, here are some books titles you might find useful:

✓ Gottman, J.M., & Schwartz Gottman, J. (2007). *And baby makes three*. New York: Three Rivers Press.

✓ Haines, S. (2007). *Healing sex*. San Francisco, CA: Cleis Press.

✓ Simkin, P., & Klaus, P. (2004). *When survivors give birth*. Seattle, WA: Classic Day Publishing.

✓ Winks, C., & Semans, A. (2004). *Sexy mamas: Keeping your sex life alive while raising kids*. Maui, HI: Inner Ocean Publishing, Inc.

✓ **Lastly, consider how you are treating your own being when working with the family.**

> This modeling goes a long way. For instance, if you are going to hold the baby, you may say out loud, "I am going to move over to pick you up from this angle, because it is better for my back," or, "Oh, let's see, I think I will sit on the bed to change your diaper, rather than lean over, because I will feel a little better that way." Here you would be modeling taking care of your body. A body that feels tended to is much more open to feeling pleasure (like hugs or gentle touch) than a body that has been neglected.

It's wonderful that you are interested in supporting the new mother. Your acknowledgment of the need for support, time, and space as she evolves in her whole being, including her sexuality, will surely go a long way.

Other Voices: Nurturing the Family's Contributing Authors

Understanding Dynamics of Oppression, Power and Privilege When Supporting Families by Naima Black

Naima Black is a full-spectrum doula, a childbirth and reproductive health educator, certified lactation counselor, and a community activist. She has supported pregnant and parenting women and their families throughout her life, including on the island of Lamu, Kenya, where she lived for 21 years. A prison rights activist and founder of Philadelphia's Maternity Care Coalition's Community Doula and Breastfeeding Program, she is also an internationally renowned Swahili interpreter.

The Business Side of Doula Work by Patty Brennan

Patty Brennan is a DONA International approved birth and postpartum doula trainer and author of *The Doula Business Guide: Creating a Successful MotherBaby Business*, 2nd Edition, and *The Doula Business Guide Workbook: Tools to Create a Thriving Business*, available through her website (www.center4cby.com) and from Amazon. In addition, she offers Small Business Basics Online, a series of eight self-paced online classes, as well as interactive Advanced Business Trainings through Center for the Childbearing Year [www.center4cby.com] in Ann Arbor, Michigan.

The Post-Baby Body: Awareness and Care by Anne Duch

Anne is a Board-Certified Women's Health Specialist and owner of Physical Therapy for Women. She is also the mom of three humans and one four-legged furry friend.

Postpartum and Sexuality by Natashia Fuksman, MA, MFT

Natashia, licensed marriage and family therapist has developed niche expertise in sex therapy, the perinatal period, and parenting in her work with individuals, couples, and families over the past 30 years. Her approach is both feminist and multicultural, stemming from her upbringing as a first-generation American woman with a multicultural, multilingual family roots. Natashia lives and works in the Bay Area offering therapy, workshops, and trainings. She has been a featured writer and speaker in several publications, podcasts, movies, and blogs, including the documentary film, *The Business of Being Born* and book, *The Ultimate Guide to Sex Through Pregnancy and Motherhood*. She is currently working on her own writing and research about the sexual development, which takes place for mothers and partners during the perinatal period. You can find out more about Natashia's offerings at www.natashiamft.com

Supporting Families through the Adoption Process and Supporting Families through the Surrogacy Process by Laura Furniss

Laura Furniss is a certified birth, bereavement, and adoption doula, who has assisted many adoptive and birth families through the birth and postpartum process. She is also a counselor who specializes in adoption, pregnancy, infertility, and pregnancy loss. When she is not assisting clients in birth and postpartum or counseling clients in life transitions and challenges, she enjoys spending time with her husband, four children through adoption, and two grandbabies.

Sensitivity: The Source of a Doula's Magic by Amy Gilliland

Amy L. Gilliland, Ph.D., AdvCD/BDT(DONA), CSE (AASECT) is a research fellow at the University of Wisconsin-Madison, one of the first DONA International birth doula trainers, an adult sexuality educator, and an infant mental health expert with specialized training in attachment. Her work has been published in multiple peer-reviewed journals and in her new book, *The Heart of the Doula: Essentials for Practice and Life*.

Loss and Grief by Ann Grauer

Ann Grauer, AdvPCD/PDT(DONA), AdvBD/BDT(DONA), LCCE, FACCE, IBCLC has worked with expectant and new families for more than 30 years. The 2007 recipient of Lamaze International's Elisabeth Bing Award, Ann has worked in various settings and has run new parents groups for 26 years. She knows that every parent has the ability to make choices that are right for themselves and their families.

The Voices of Birdsong Brooklyn by Laura Interlandi and Erica Livingston

Erica Livingston and Laura Interlandi are doulas, writers, mentors, and co-founders of Birdsong Brooklyn. Together, they teach in person and through their online Learning Lodge. They have known and loved Jackie since 2013, quote her almost daily, and believe deeply in the power of tethering together to mentors, mentees, and those they serve to support each other's highest dreams and visions. You can find them at birdsongbrooklyn.com.

Possibilities: When Life Includes a Family Member with a Disability by Jamie Lee Marks

Jamie Lee Marks is a certified vision rehabilitation therapist and inclusive education teacher. Jamie has over 25 years teaching individuals of all ages, stages, and possibilities. Along with her faithful seeing-eye canine, Frenchie, Jamie lives with her husband, Michael, and they have two big kids.

Supporting LGBTQ Families in the Postpartum by Morgane Richardson

Morgane Richardson has been doula and perinatal health educator since 2012 and wears a variety of hats in this field, including Former Director of the NYC Doula Collective and Founder of Woven Bodies, an inclusive digital practice supporting queer folks + allies from family planning through parenthood. Morgane's reflections on gender, race, and sexuality have been published in numerous media outlets including BirthFit Podcast, Doula International, and InsideOut. Morgane makes her home in Brooklyn, NY with her wife Alexandra and their daughter, Woolf Rose.

The Transition to Dadhood by Dr. Jay Warren

Dr. Jay Warren is a prenatal and pediatric chiropractor in San Diego, where he works with new families every day. Dr. Jay is the host of two popular podcasts, "Healthy Births, Happy Babies" and "The Dadhood Journey," as well as an instructor for the ICPA (International Chiropractic Pediatric Association). He is also the proud father to his son, Niko, who inspires him to strive to be a better person and better dad every day.

References

Bateson, M.C. (2001). *Composing a life.* Grove Press.

Brown, B. (2015). *Daring greatly: How the courage to be vulnerable transforms the way we live, love, parent, and lead.* New York: Penguin Randomhouse.

Cronwett, L. (1985). Parental network structure and perceived support after birth of first child. *Nursing Research,* 34(6), 347-352.

Dekker, R. (2017). Evidence on IV fluids during labor. Retrieved from https://evidencebasedbirth.com/iv-fluids-during-labor/

DONA International. (2016). Position appear: The postpartum doula's role in maternity care. Retrieved from https://www.dona.org/wp-content/uploads/2018/03/DONA-Postpartum-Position-Paper-FINAL.pdf

Godin, S. (2008). *Tribes: We need you to lead us.* New York: Penguin Group.

Gold, M. (1990). *Try another way.* Marc Gold and Associates.

Hartley, G. (2018). *Fed up: Emotional labor, women, and the way forward.* New York: HarperCollins Publishers.

Ilse, S. (1996). *Giving care, taking care: Support for the helpers.* Wintergreen Press.

Katherine, A. (1994) *Boundaries: Where you end and I begin—How to recognize and set healthy boundaries.* Hazelden Publishing.

Klaus, M., & Klaus, P. (2001). *Your amazing newborn.* DaCapo Lifelong Books.

Olson, Haider et al. (2010). A quasi-medical evaluation of a breastfeeding support program for low-income women in Michigan. *Maternal Child Health Journal,* 14, 86-93.

Ou, H. (2016). *The first forty days: The essential art of nourishing the new mother.* Harry N. Abrams.

Ruiz, D.M. (1997). *The four agreements: A practical guide to personal freedom (A Toltec Wisdom Book).* California, Amber-Allen Publishing.

Simkin, P. (1991). Just another day in a woman's life? Women's long-term perceptions of their first birth experience. Part 1. *Birth, 18(4),* 203-210.

Simkin, P. (2019). *Birth trauma: Definition and statistics.* Retrieved from Wolman, W. et al (1993). Postpartum depression and companionship in the clinical birth environment: A randomized, controlled study. *American Journal of Obstetrics and Gynecology,* 163, 1388-1393.

About the Author

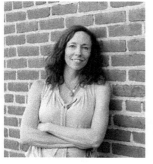

Jacqueline Kelleher began supporting families as a doula in 1993, working under the title, "I help out when people have babies." That's still pretty accurate today, although extensive training and certifications entitles her to use the more official-sounding doula, childbirth educator and lactation counselor.

In the years that followed, Jacqueline became a professional birth doula and doula trainer. In 2002 she became DONA's Director of Postpartum Services and cofounder of their postpartum certification program. For twelve years, she served with the organization's leadership as a board member and as program mentor. She has supported thousands of families as well as thousands of doulas. Every family and every individual she has worked with and for has been a teacher and their lessons are woven into the offerings within these pages.

Jacqueline's family is the foundation of her drive to support. Personal experiences with support—both its presence and its absence—shaped her expectations of what life can and should offer families. She has three grown, wonderful children, and one much younger, equally as wonderful, still at home. She has been hands-on "mom"-ing for 28 years.

The other focus of her life has been the study of martial arts and self-defense. She is a third degree black belt and a retired instructor. While these may seem divergent fields, she finds constant intersections. Finding voice, making choices, setting boundaries, and feeling amazed by the power of what our bodies can do; the two are related more often than not.

CPSIA information can be obtained
at www.ICGtesting.com
Printed in the USA
BVHW050819260223
659230BV00013B/750